EARLY DETECTION OF BREAST CANCER

Risk, Detection Protocols, and Therapeutic Implications

John K. Gohagan et al.

Library of Congress Cataloging in Publication Data
Main entry under title:

Early detection of breast cancer.

    Bibliography: p.
    Includes index.
    1. Breast — Cancer — Diagnosis. 2. Breast —
Radiography. I. Gohagan, John K. [DNLM:
1. Breast neoplasms. WP 870 E118]
RC280.B8E23   616.99′449075   81-17884
ISBN 0-03-059389-1   AACR2

Published in 1982 by Praeger Publishers
CBS Educational and Professional Publishing
a Division of CBS Inc.
521 Fifth Avenue, New York, New York 10175 U.S.A.

© 1982 by Praeger Publishers

23456789 145 987654321

Printed in the United States of America

THE AUTHORS

John K. Gohagan, Ph.D., Principal Investigator
Associate Professor, Preventive Medicine
Associate Professor, Engineering and Applied Science
Director, Division of Health Care Research in Preventive Medicine
Washington University, St. Louis, Missouri

Ned D. Rodes, M.D., Co-Principal Investigator
Director, Breast Cancer Detection Demonstration Project No. 25
Cancer Research Center, Columbia, Missouri

Walter F. Ballinger, M.D.
Professor, Surgery
Washington University, St. Louis, Missouri

Charles W. Blackwell, M.D.
Radiologist, Breast Cancer Detection Demonstration Project No. 25
Cancer Research Center, Columbia, Missouri

Harvey R. Butcher, M.D.
Professor, Surgery
Washington University, St. Louis, Missouri

William P. Darby, Ph.D.
Associate Professor, Engineering and Applied Science
Washington University, St. Louis, Missouri

Dinah K. Pearson, B.A.
Coordinator, Breast Cancer Detection Demonstration Project No. 25
Cancer Research Center, Columbia, Missouri

Edward L. Spitznagel, Ph.D.
Professor, Mathematics
Washington University, St. Louis, Missouri

Marc K. Wallack, M.D.
Assistant Professor, Surgery
Washington, University, St. Louis, Missouri

PREFACE

In 1976 a graduate student, Rita Menitoff, and I began an analysis of the literature on the early detection of breast cancer. We organized published data for use in an elementary decision model for evaluating detection protocols and individual detection modalities in common use. We concluded our critique of the literature nearly a year later with the realization that the data available in the literature could not be used with any confidence to evaluate and compare detection protocols. For this purpose we needed detection data from a screening project where a large number of asymptomatic women had been screened periodically for a number of years, where the same detection modalities were applied independently to each woman, where the detection data were accurately and consistently collected and stored, and where case follow-up was an integral part of the program.

Walter Ballinger and Harvey Butcher, surgeons at Washington University, provided essential assistance at this point by introducing me to Ned Rodes, a surgeon at the Cancer Research Center in Columbia, Missouri, who was directing one of the national Breast Cancer Detection Demonstration Projects (BCDDPs) sponsored by the National Cancer Institute and the American Cancer Society. The data base at this screening project was as close an approximation to our needs as we could expect to find. Mutual interest led to a research partnership that made it possible for us to evaluate and compare Xerox mammography, thermography, and clinical palpation as individual modalities and in multimodality protocols for screening asymptomatic women.

In 1979 the National Center for Health Services Research provided funding (Grant No. R01HS3256) to continue the mathematical modeling effort and to evaluate the detection modalities using screening data from BCDDP No. 25. Other support was provided by the American Cancer Society (Grant No. IN-36-R), by the Public Health Service (Institutional Biomedical Research Support Grant), and by the Cancer Research Center.

This book is the product of nearly four years of work by a multidisciplinary group of scientists and physicians. The entire effort has been a most rewarding experience and the results are important.

John K. Gohagan

ACKNOWLEDGMENTS

Many people have contributed to the years of effort that preceded the preparation of this book. Radiologist Corinne Farrell, M.D. read all thermograms. William Short, Deborah Wallace, and Victor Conocchioli carried the burden of initial data coding, which took many months. Timothy Herder, Joseph Feiner, Thomas Frank, and Carlene Walters assisted with statistical computing and data management. Valjean Spear contributed successfully to strategy enumeration. Rita Menitoff conducted an excellent critique of the literature on breast cancer detection and therapy, as did John Goodman of the recent literature on risk profiling. Lillian Beal and Phyllis Anderson typed the manuscript, and Linda Beck helped coordinate manuscript production. Alice Clarke did the art work. And Brenda Matthews, R.T.; Linda Grotewiel, R.N.; Dorothy Treaster; Margaret Woodruff; Shirley Stewart; Betty Black, R.N.; Rosetta Miller, R.N.; Patti Burton; Shelley Brandenburg, R.N.; Dixie Speer; Ginger Crain Mesks; Marjorie Baskett; Pauline Donaldson; Mike Callais; Avis Marshall; Margaret Cutts, M.T.; Marsha Howard, R.T.; Jo Moran, R.N.; and others helped make this study possible by their work on BCDDP No. 25.

CONTENTS

x

1

INTRODUCTION

John K. Gohagan

Breast cancer is one of the most serious diseases threatening U.S. women today. More than 90,000 new cases of breast cancer are diagnosed annually. It is the leading cause of cancer deaths among women between 40 and 49 years of age [Mueller et al. 1978]. The New York Health Insurance Plan (HIP) study showed survival advantages resulting from early detection of breast cancer among women 50 years of age or older [Shapiro et al. 1974]. And there is rather widespread belief that similar advantages may accrue to younger women, even though they were not evident in the HIP study.

This book is about early detection of breast cancer in asymptomatic women. We address three major questions:

How accurate are individual detection modalities in a screening environment?

Which multimodality protocols are best for women of high, medium, and low risk?

What is the risk-benefit balance for X-ray mammography, and how often should mammograms be scheduled?

We use screening data from Breast Cancer Detection Demonstration Project (BCDDP) No. 25 to evaluate modality accuracy in that setting. We use these data in conjunction with cost data to determine optimal and suboptimal multimodality detection strategies for women by risk level. But BCDDP data cannot be used in the risk-benefit analysis because there is no information in that data base that could be used to calculate potential X-radiation risk. Hence, national and international epidemiological data plus economic factors form the basis for this effort.

The problem of risk profiling with epidemiological variables such as family history with breast cancer, reproductive history, and chronological age is discussed briefly. Epidemiological data from BCDDP No. 25 are analyzed via multivariate statistical techniques, and the generally insignificant results raise serious doubts about the possibility of developing useful multivariate risk profiles from medical history data.

The book is organized into three parts. Part I documents the screening process at BCDDP No. 25 and presents basic statistics contrasting it with the other 26 BCDDPs in aggregate and, to a limited extent, with breast cancer detection practices in other kinds of clinical settings. The purpose of this part is to give the reader a perspective for judging the quality of the BCDDP No. 25 data base. Part II contains all the analytical chapters and begins with an encapsulated discussion of the analytical methods employed. Subsequent chapters address the issues of risk profiling, modality evaluation, protocol or strategy selection, the risk-benefit balance for mammography, and examination scheduling. Part III contains two chapters covering the clinical implications of our findings and the therapeutic implications of early detection.

Economic questions are central to the analysis presented in Part II and to our final conclusions. This is a fairly complex topic since there is quite a bit of variability in detection and treatment costs in different settings and because psychosocial costs in the form of what economists call opportunity costs are necessarily included. Cost data and estimation techniques are presented in Appendix B.

This book is also about analytical technique. The entire research effort could be categorized as applied systems analysis or operations research in a field recently labeled clinical epidemiology. With the increasing interest of mathematical scientists in medical decision making and the concomitant interest of a small group of physicians in statistical decision theory, one can expect to see many more studies of this type. Consideration of the methodology of our study should be useful to other analysts. In particular an original decision analytic tool for evaluating multistage decision problems is illustrated in the chapter on strategy evaluation.

REFERENCES

Mueller CD, Ames F, Anderson GD (1978) Breast cancer in 3,558 women: age as a significant determinant in rate of dying and causes of death. Surgery 83:123–131.

Shapiro S, Strax P, Venet L, Venet W (1974) Changes in 5-year breast cancer mortality in a breast cancer screening program, *in* Seventh National Cancer Conference Proceedings, pp. 663–678. Washington, D.C., American Cancer Society, January 1974.

PART I

Screening at BCDDP NO. 25

The screening data used in this book are from the medical records of 10,187 initially asymptomatic women screened at least annually at Breast Cancer Detection Demonstration Project (BCDDP) No. 25 in Columbia, Missouri. Epidemiological and financial data used in the study came from a variety of other sources including published reports and hospital records. BCDDP data are used only to evaluate detection modalities in that screening environment.

The screening process and summary statistics for BCDDP No. 25 are presented in this part. The data collection forms completed by examiners and some additional information specific to BCDDPs are included in Appendix A.

2

Data and Summary Statistics
for BCDDP NO. 25

Dinah K. Pearson
Ned D. Rodes
Charles W. Blackwell
John K. Gohagan

In 1973 the National Cancer Institute (NCI) in cooperation with the American Cancer Society (ACS) initiated, with congressional encouragement, the National Breast Cancer Detection Demonstration Project (NBCDDP). The NBCDDP was designed initially not as a research project but as a mechanism for conveying in practice and in concept the benefits of screening, as projected from the New York Health Insurance Plan (HIP) experiences of the 1960s, to the adult female population of the nation. As initially conceived, the immediate objectives were to test in practice the enthusiasm of asymptomatic women for regular periodic breast examinations and to demonstrate to the medical profession the usefulness of regular screening for early detection of breast cancer. Education of both the public and the medical profession was of prime concern.

By 1975, 27 individual screening projects (BCDDPs) were established around the nation (Table 2.1). Each had recruited a participating population of about 10,000 asymptomatic women 35 years of age and older for free annual screening by medical history, physical examination, X-ray mammography, and heat-sensing thermography during the five-year screening project. In addition to screening, participants were to receive five years of follow-up inquiry on their health status beginning in the sixth year of participation. Funding was provided via NCI contracts and ACS grants with budgets between approximately $200,000 and $400,000 annually. Overall NBCDDP management was provided by NCI.

Although standardized screening and data collection practices were not required of BCDDPs initially, NCI increasingly tightened its guidelines. By 1974 NBCDDP guidelines had evolved substantially as indicated in the

TABLE 2.1.
BCDDP Locations

Ann Arbor, Mich.	Nashville, Tenn.
Atlanta, Ga.	New York, N.Y.
Boise, Idaho	Newark, N.J.
Cincinnati, Ohio	Oakland, Calif.
Columbia, Mo.	Oklahoma City, Okla.
Des Moines, Iowa	Philadelphia, Pa.*
Durham, N.C.	Pittsburgh, Pa.
Honolulu, Hawaii	Portland, Oreg.
Houston, Tex.	Providence, R.I.
Jacksonville, Fla.	Seattle, Wash.
Kansas City, Kans.	Tucson, Ariz.
Los Angeles, Calif.	Washington, D.C.
Louisville, Ky.	Wilmington, Del.
Milwaukee, Wis.	

*There were two centers in both Atlanta and Philadelphia. Each city had a total of 10,000 participants, except New York City which had 20,000.

"Informed Consent Record" that appears in Appendix A. A requirement of independent diagnostic testing (including test interpretation) was specified for newly funded BCDDPs. Standardized data collection forms were being adopted by all BCDDPs [HEW/PHS/NIH 1978]. Thus data from BCDDPs funded in 1974 had substantial potential for systematic evaluation of individual detection modalities and multimodality protocols.

BCDDP NO. 25

Funding for BCDDP No. 25 at the Cancer Research Center in Columbia, Missouri, was awarded in March 1974. The contract was signed and screening actually began in June 1974. Participants were recruited from 105 of Missouri's 115 counties. Recruiting mechanisms included an ACS volunteer recruiter in each of 21 mid-Missouri counties, special news releases by the Cancer Research Center for television, radio, and newspapers, and physician/patient interaction. About 5,000 women were screened in the first year of operation, and a full complement of 10,187 asymptomatic women between the ages of 35 and 74 years had been accepted and screened by April 1976.

Demographic statistics for the population screened at BCDDP No. 25 are given in Table 2.2. This is a rather homogeneous population that is slightly older, more rural, and less wealthy than participating populations at other BCDDPs. Owing to the effort put forth by project staff, participation

TABLE 2.2.
Demographic Facts for BCDDP No. 25 Participants

	BCDDP No. 25	NBCDDP Average
Number of participants	10,187	10,000
Protestant religion	84 percent	58 percent
Race	97 percent	87 percent
Average age		
Overall at initial exam	52 years	49 years
Cancer patients	59 years	Unknown
Family income ≤ $15,000	64 percent	49 percent
Married or widowed	94 percent	88 percent
Some college training	37 percent	44 percent
Initially asymptomatic*	100 percent	Unknown
Missouri counties represented	105 of 115, including St. Louis City	n.a.

n.a. = not applicable

*Although all women were technically asymptomatic when they entered the program, 124 had had a previous mastectomy. Nine of these women developed cancer in the remaining breast. Six of these women suffered chest wall recurrences.

continuity was greater than at the other BCDDPs, as shown by the comparative continuation rates in Table 2.3.

SCREENING AND DATA COLLECTION PRACTICES AT BCDDP NO. 25

BCDDP No. 25 staff strictly adhered to a scientific protocol designed to permit comparative evaluations of the individual detection modalities and multimodality strategies. Detailed medical histories were taken by ACS volunteers at the initial visit and updated at each subsequent visit. Each of the examiners functioned independently of all others. None had access to

TABLE 2.3.
Continuity of Participation

Period	Percentage Rescreened	
	BCDDP No. 25	NBCDDP Average*
Year 2	95.6	85.2
Year 3	89.7	73.9
Year 4	89.0	67.0
Year 5	83.6	62.8

*Data Management Center Report 1/7/81.

TABLE 2.4.
Variables Coded for Computer Analysis

HISTORY

Date. Visit number. Age
Months since last exam
Current breast problems
Age at menarche
Age at first pregnancy

Months since last exam
Family incidence of breast cancer
Current hormone consumption
Number of live births
Number of unsuccessful pregnancies

Number previous X rays
Previous breast biopsy
Age of menopause
Age at first birth
Total months of breast feeding

THERMOGRAPHY

Date. Visit number
Asymmetric areolar temperatures
Diagnosis

Asymmetric background temperatures
Side(s) of increased temperature
Recommendations

Asymmetric vascular patterns
Confidence of examiner

MAMMOGRAPHY

Date. Visit number
Nipple changes
Marginal characteristics of masses
Distribution of calcifications
Diagnosis

Breast sizes
Number of masses
Shapes of masses
Shapes of calcifications
Recommendations

Skin changes
Locations of (dominant and other) masses
Dimensions of masses
Locations of architectural distortions
Confidence of examiner

PHYSICAL EXAMINATION

Date. Visit number
Texture of dominant mass
Nodularity of breasts
Skin changes
Diagnosis

Locations of masses
Mobility of dominant mass
Thickening of breasts
Palpable axillary nodes
Recommendations

Dimensions of dominant mass
Shape of dominant mass
Nipple changes
Retraction of breast
Confidence of examiner

FINAL SCREENING REVIEW

Date. Visit number

Modality reinterpretation

Final recommendations

Note: Detailed subdivisions — as, for example, those specifying which family members had breast cancer — are not shown but are included in the computerized data base.

any information about a participant from other tests as a basis for interpretation. The nurse practitioners who conducted all clinical examinations had access to the medical history forms as well as to facts provided by screenees during the examination. The mammographer knew the age of the screenee and compared previous X-rays with current X-rays in the interpretation process. The thermographer saw only the thermograms. Screening began wth thermography, followed by mammography and subsequently by clinical examination. Thermography was done first to avoid spurious heat patterns generated in the process of the other tests. Nearly all mammograms were read by a single radiologist. All thermograms were read by another radiologist.

For the first four years all participants underwent all three procedures at regular annual screenings.[1] However, the techniques were selectively employed when women were recalled for early reexamination on the basis of suspicious findings. Using only their own test information, each examiner independently formulated an interpretation and recommended a course of action. The mammographer and clinicians could recommend tissue biopsy, aspiration, early recall for reexamination, or review of the case by the entire examining team. The physician-thermographer was constrained from recommending either biopsy or aspiration—because abnormal readings on thermography were common with benign disease—but could indicate suspicion of malignancy and ask for review of the case. In no case was a final-screening recommendation made other than routine annual rescreening, except on the basis of a case-review conference in which all examiners participated. These conferences were held approximately once each week; and at conference the observations, interpretations, and recommendations of all examiners were reviewed in the light of all medicohistorical data in a woman's medical file.

Standard forms used for data collection are included in Appendix A. Most of the data were coded for computer analysis. The major variables included in our computerized data base are summarized in Table 2.4. Each visit by a participant translated into ten 80-column cards of data covering medical history, the findings on all three tests, final recommendations for further action on behalf of a screenee, and pathology for diagnostic and therapeutic surgery, when appropriate.

SUMMARY STATISTICS

More than 50,000 visits were completed during the five-year screening program. On screening, 644 biopsy recommendations were made.[2] Of these, 576 were completed and pathology evaluations for all were recorded. Over 257 additional biopsies were performed on participating women in the intervals between screenings that were not on the basis of BCDDP screening results. The pathologies of these, too, were recorded. Recommended biopsies yielded 136 cancer cases, while interval biopsies yielded 16 for a total of 152 cancers in five years. Yield in terms of total cancers found to total biopsies was about 6.2 percent (16/257) for interval biopsies and 23.6 percent (136/576) for screening. The age distribution for cancers detected was: 35 to 44 years, 7.2 percent; 45 to 54 years, 27 percent; 55 to 64 years, 33.6 percent; and 65 years or older, 32.2 percent.

Of the 152 cancers 59 were discovered during the (participant's) first year in the project, 30 cases in the second year, 19 in the third year, 26 in the fourth, and 18 in the fifth and final year. Corresponding approximate prevalence and incidence rates for the population were 6/1,000, 3/1,000, 2/1,000, 3/1,000 and 2/1,000, respectively.[3] The high prevalence rate is above the average reported in the literature, is typical of BCDDPs, and probably reflects two facts, namely, that the screening population was largely self-selecting and possibly at high risk and that BCDDP No. 25 detected proportionately more early cancers than the average clinic.

The 152 cancers represent 148 women. Nine of the women had had cancer diagnosed in the opposite breast prior to joining the project. One woman had cancers detected simultaneously in both breasts. And three women had cancer detected subsequently in the opposite breast.

Of the 136 cancers detected in screening, mammography identified 86 percent and clinical palpation identified 44 percent. Mammography alone detected 56 percent of the cancers, while palpation alone detected 14 percent of them. In 89 percent of those detected by mammography alone no axillary lymph nodes were found positive on pathology, while for clinical palpation the corresponding number is 63 percent. Overall 105 (77 percent) of cases detected on screening had negative axillary lymph nodes.

Screening yield in terms of cancers detected per 100 biopsies improved from the 18 in the first year of operation to 36 in the fifth year with most of the gain in the first two years as the medical staff became ever more capable of discriminating between malignant and benign disease on the basis of test information [Gohagan et al. 1980].

More than 44 percent of the 76 cancerous tumors detected on screening for which size was recorded were 1 cm or less in diameter. This compares quite favorably with national data showing 30 to 35 percent and reflects the power of high quality mammography to detect small lesions [Working Group Report 1977].

NOTES

1. After September 1977 mammography was restricted to women over 50 years of age with certain exceptions. The 50-year age limit did not apply when a woman's personal physician requested mammography, when a palpable mass was present, when there was a history of cancer in the opposite breast, or when a woman was over 40 years old and her mother and/or sister had a history of breast cancer. True positive and true negative rates calculated from

BCDDP No. 25 data are not influenced by this policy change because the conclusions are based on only those screens (nearly 40,000) for which all modalities were applied.

2. BCDDPs screen only. It is up to a woman's personal physician to act on BCDDP biopsy recommendations. BCDDP No. 25 staff actively pursued cases for compliance. More than 90% of the recommended biopsies were performed.

3. *Prevalence* is the rate of cancers in a previously unscreened population. *Incidence* is the rate at which new cancers are generated in a population. First-year rates for BCDDP No. 25 are close to true prevalence, while third- through fifth-year rates are close to true incidence in the population. The second-year rate is a mix of prevalence cancers undetected in the first year and new clinically occult cancers that developed between the first and second screening.

REFERENCES

Gohagan JK, Rodes ND, Blackwell CW, Darby WP, Farrell C, Herder TJ, Pearson DK, Spitznagel EL, Wallace D (1980) Individual and combined effectiveness of palpation, thermography, and mammography in breast cancer screening. Preventive Medicine 9:713–721.

Report of the Working Group to Review the NCI-ACS Breast Cancer Detection Demonstration Projects (1977), Vol. 1, Special Report Section A. Bethesda, Md., National Cancer Institute.

Rodes ND, Farrell C, Blackwell CW (1977) Missouri's role in breast cancer detection. Missouri Medicine, pp. 689–694.

U.S., Department of Health, Education and Welfare/Public Health Service/National Institutes of Health (1978) Manual of Procedures and Operations for the National Cancer Institute and the American Cancer Society Breast Cancer Detection Demonstration Project. Washington, D.C., USDHEW.

3

Mammography

Charles W. Blackwell

The mammogram has been the major factor in earlier detection of breast disease during the past two decades. Evidence from the New York Health Insurance Plan (HIP) study and more recently from the Breast Cancer Detection Demonstration Projects (BCDDPs) has showed that good quality mammography is the most important modality for detecting clinically occult breast cancer. Not only is mammography capable of detecting preclinical lesions, it is also beneficial in the differential diagnosis of clinically evident or questionable breast abnormalities.

This chapter will briefly deal with the technique of Xerox mammography and primarily with the radiographic interpretation.

TECHNIQUE

Mammography may be accomplished with either film or Xerox techniques. Either form, using good technique, will produce high quality diagnostic images. Some radiologists prefer film, some prefer Xerox, while a few advise both techniques. At the Cancer Research Center (CRC) in Columbia, Missouri, the Xerox process is used exclusively. We have found it to be a highly reliable technique and, in addition, prefer it because of its speed and ease of interpretation. This becomes even more important in a busy X-ray department or screening center where large volumes of examinations must be interpreted.

At the CRC two views are routine: the recumbent mediolateral and the cephalocaudad projection. Occasionally, additional views such as lateromedial, contact, axillary, "cleopatra" views of the axillary tail, rotated cephalocaudad, or dependent cephalocaudad views may be necessary.

Compression of the breast is very important and is always done in the routine mediolateral and cephalocaudad views. This is done with a balloon in the end of the X-ray mammographic cone. Compression changes the usual conical shape of the breast to a more uniform thickness, thus allowing radiographic imaging of the entire breast from the thicker portion, near the chest wall, to the nipple, all in one lateral view. The wide latitude of the Xerox process facilitates this. Compression also diminishes scatter radiation—and possibly motion—and thus also helps to produce better resolution. Using one-second exposure times, motion is the most common cause of poor quality images.

It is extremely important that the entire breast be viewed on the mediolateral projection. Otherwise, lesions near the chest wall may be missed. It is impossible to view the entire breast tissue adjacent to the chest wall on the cephalocaudad projection. For this reason it is preferable that the lateral views be done recumbent, with a wedge of sponge between the breast and Xerox cassette to push the lateral axillary portion anteriorly away from the chest wall and into the path of the X-ray beam—and thus take an image of the entire breast from chest wall to nipple. At times it is preferable not to use the wedge sponge. Slightly better resolution may be obtained without the sponge, thus decreasing the "target-film" distance by putting the breast in contact with the Xerox cassette. However, the posterior portion of the breast next to the chest wall and especially the axillary portion of the breast cannot be imaged in this fashion. Some mammographers prefer that two mediolateral views be obtained, one with the sponge, viewing the entire breast and chest wall, and the other without the sponge (a contact mediolateral), producing slightly better resolution at the cost of not viewing the entire breast. Usually, resolution is adequate with the sponge, and only rarely is a contact view necessary. It is much easier and faster for technicians to image the entire breast on recumbent lateral views than it is on upright lateral projections. This is of time-saving importance in a busy, large volume X-ray department or screening situation. It is too time-consuming to try to obtain good quality mediolateral views of the entire breast in the upright position.

The most frequent additional views that are necessary are the rotated or exaggerated cephalocaudad projections. Occasionally, when a lesion is noted on the lateral view near the chest wall, it may not be imaged on a routine cephalocaudad projection. Additional views should then be obtained with the breast rotated first to include more of the lateral aspect and then rotated the opposite way to include more of the medial aspect of the breast. This way most lesions can be located. Rarely, if a lesion is not localized near the chest wall in this fashion, dependent hanging cephalocaudal views may be obtained with a horizontal X-ray beam. The dependent view does not allow good diagnostic resolution but will be adequate to localize a suspicious area not seen on the other cephalocaudal views.

The technical factors utilized depend upon the target-film distance, the consistency of the breast, and whether a positive or negative mode Xerox image is desired. Either a molybdenum or tungsten target X-ray tube may be utilized; however, the skin dosage to the patient will be smaller with an image produced by a tungsten target X-ray tube. At the CRC we utilize tungsten target tubes with 1.0 mm of added aluminum filtration in the X-ray beam. This creates a half-value layer (HVL) of 1.5 mm Al. The milliamperage seconds (MAS) used depend on the length of the X-ray cone. With the single-phase Picker Mammorex unit with a tungsten target and target skin distance of 52 cm, 200 MAS is utilized for a positive mode (blue on a white background) Xerox image. For a negative mode technique (white on a blue background) 140 MAS is utilized. The kilovolt peak (KVP) utilized for a mediolateral projection on a breast of average consistency and size is in the 40 to 45 KVP range. For images produced with an ordinary rotating tungsten target X-ray tube, adapted with a long cone (target skin distance [TSD] 80 cm) utilizing the technique of Wolfe, [1972], 300 MAS is utilized for positive mode images and 200 MAS for negative mode images. This produces a skin dose of about 1.0 R to the patient for positive mode and correspondingly less for negative mode images. The midplane dose has been calculated to be about 0.25 to 0.5 R for a positive mode image in an average-sized breast. There are advantages other than lowering the dosage to the patient of the negative mode technique. Punctate calcifications seem to show up better, as does the parenchymal pattern of the breast, in some cases. The dense breast, especially the small, dense breast, is better examined by negative mode technique. However, sometimes the positive mode technique seems beneficial. At times masses seem more evident on a positive mode and at other times more evident on a negative mode image. Almost all of the original BCDDP images were made with positive mode with selected cases being done in the negative mode. More recently, the negative mode technique has been utilized more and more, and we are currently using positive mode technique for the mediolateral image and negative mode for the cephalocaudad image, thus taking advantage of each technique.

The Xerox images are mounted side to side for ease of interpretation and comparison. As a personal preference, the left breast is mounted on the right as the viewer looks at the images, and the right breast is mounted on the left as the interpreter faces the images. It is very important to view both images simultaneously since the breasts are very similar in appearance and any difference between the two should arouse some suspicion. It should also be noted that the Xerox technique produces a mirror image instead of a direct image like film mammography (the Xerox process first produces an image on a metal plate, and the image from the plate is then transferred to the Xerox paper, thus producing a mirror image). For more detail in technique and the Xerox process, the reader is referred to the excellent texts of Wolfe [1972] and Egan [1976].

MAMMOGRAPHIC INTERPRETATION

Properly mounted side by side, the images should be viewed under a very bright hi-intensity light and through a low-power hand-held magnifying lens. The images are quickly scanned for quality of technique and to determine if any additional views may be necessary. The images must be of high diagnostic quality, and if not, should be repeated. Previous mammograms, if any, should be readily available for comparison. The history and physical findings should also be available for the radiologist during interpretation.

At BCDDP No. 25 the mammograms were read without the privilege or knowledge of the history or physical examination. In practice, however, this information can at times be quite beneficial in formulating a more comprehensive X-ray report that is correlated with clinical data. A brief history concerning factors such as gravidity, parity, menstrual history, age, previous breast diseases, or biopsies, whether there has been previous breast cancer in the patient's family, and the physical findings of the breast examination should be available. Clinically palpated masses should be localized on an accompanying diagram and characterized as to their size, shape, and consistency. Also in the physical examination any unusual thickenings or other abnormalities in the breast consistency should be noted. Scars on the skin, including biopsy scars, are very important to note for the mammographer. Any skin lesions such as rashes, nevi, keloids, accessory nipples, or any other skin abnormalities should be noted. If the above information concerning the history and physical is not available to the mammographer, then his technicians should be taught to take a brief history concerning the factors outlined above and to examine the patients. Some mammographers prefer to do the physical exam themselves, and this should certainly be done if a reliable physical exam report is not available to the mammographer. A much more knowledgeable interpretation and better service to the patient and her physician can be rendered by the mammographer if the history and physical can be correlated with mammographic interpretation.

The primary mammographic abnormalities to be noted are masses, calcification, architectural distortion, nonspecific areas of increased density, dilated ducts, and developing densities.

Masses

Most benign masses are round or oval with smooth, sharply demarcated margins. (Figs. 3.1–3.38 provide examples of various types of malignant and nonmalignant masses.) They are usually cysts or fibroadenomas and have the same radiographic density. These cannot be differentiated with certainty on the mammogram except when a fibroadenoma degenerates and becomes calcified. Usually, the type of calcification in a degenerated fibroadenoma is characteristic and of the large popcorn-type variety. Other lesions that would have to be considered in the differential diagnosis would be fibrolipomas (pure lipomas are radiolucent), fat necrosis, hematomas, or intramammary lymph nodes. Rarely, a malignant tumor may have a benign appearance and be fairly well circumscribed with a smooth margin. Medullary carcinoma, mucoid carcinoma, tubular carcinoma, and, infrequently, ordinary infiltrating ductal carcinoma may be well circumscribed, and very rarely a carcinoma may occur within a cyst. Cystosarcoma phylloides is well circumscribed and smooth or lobulated in outline, and we have seen two examples of plasmacytomas, which are well circumscribed. Some metastatic lesions may also be fairly round and smooth and may have a "benign" radiographic appearance.

The malignant masses are usually irregular, and their margins may be stellate, nodular, spiculated, indistinct, or lobulated in character. Often times, a breast mass is only partially visualized, being partially obscured by dense overlying breast parenchyma. Even if the visualized portion of the breast mass is round and smooth, its benignity cannot be guaranteed on the mammogram. If a portion of the mass margin is indistinct, it would have to be considered indeterminant and either aspiration, ultrasound, or biopsy considered. And, as noted in the preceding paragraph, rarely, a completely seen benign-appearing, round, smooth mass may be, indeed, malignant. Conversely, all masses that are not round and smooth are not necessarily malignant. Mammary dysplasia frequently produces irregular conglomerate mass-like densities. It is quite helpful to note whether there are any punctate calcifications since approximately 50 percent of breast carcinomas will have some of these punctate calcifications, which when present will therefore increase the degree of suspicion.

Calcifications

Calcifications are frequent in the breast, and they occur in benign and malignant disease. The types of calcification that occur in the breast are punctate (tiny pinpoint dots or like small thin grains of sand), ringlike (doughnut shaped), linear (or rodlike), and conglomerate (popcorn-like shaped). The calcification may be distributed or arranged in various fashions. The punctate calcification may be diffusely scattered throughout the entire breast or a segment. They may be sparsely or heavily concentrated. Or they may be grouped closely in tight clusters of a few or innumerable punctate calcifications. It is the clustering together of these

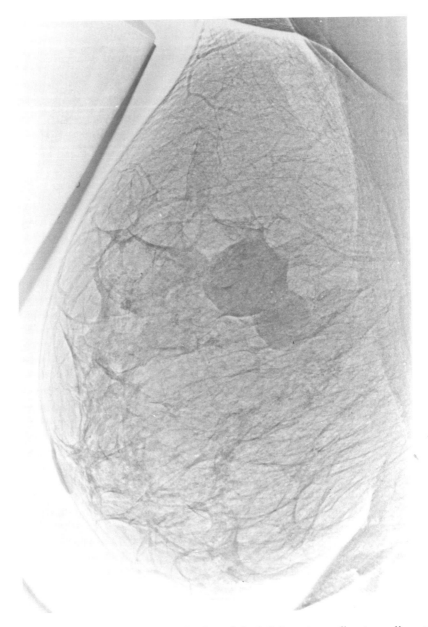

Fig. 3.1. A mediolateral projection of the left breast revealing two adjacent round uncalcified masses. The anterior margins on each of the masses are round, smooth, and sharply demarcated, having a classically benign appearance. However, the posterior margin of the inferior mass is indistinct, and the margin of the superior mass posteriorly is somewhat irregular. Although these are most likely benign, it would be recommended that ultrasound, aspiration, or biopsy be utilized to help confirm this impression. If the densities prove to be cystic on ultrasound and/or aspiration, nothing further need be done. If the lesions prove to be solid on ultrasound or if aspiration were unsuccessful or bloody or had positive cytology, then excision would be recommended. Both of these were cysts.

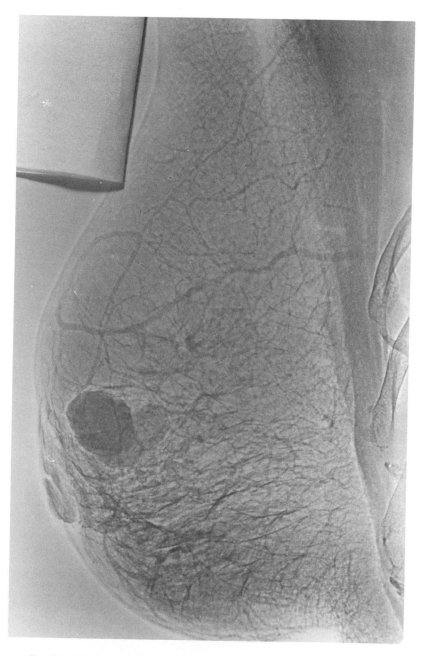

Fig. 3.2. The left mediolateral projection is somewhat similar to Fig. 3.1, with three adjacent masses that are most likely benign; similar management would be indicated as for the case in Fig. 3.1. A well-circumscribed lobulated neoplasm may rarely produce an appearance similar to this. No calcifications are evident in the masses. These also were cysts.

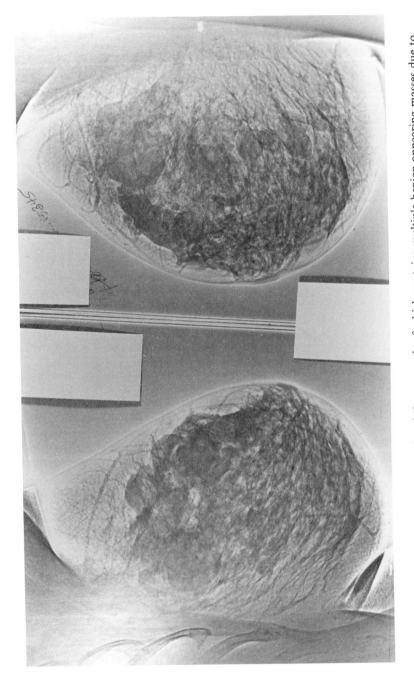

Fig. 3.3. The lateral projections of each breast, each of which contains multiple benign-appearing masses due to extensive bilateral cystic disease. The margins of many of these lesions are partially obscured by overlying dense breast parenchyma and other masses. It is, therefore, impossible to be certain that all of the masses are benign in nature.

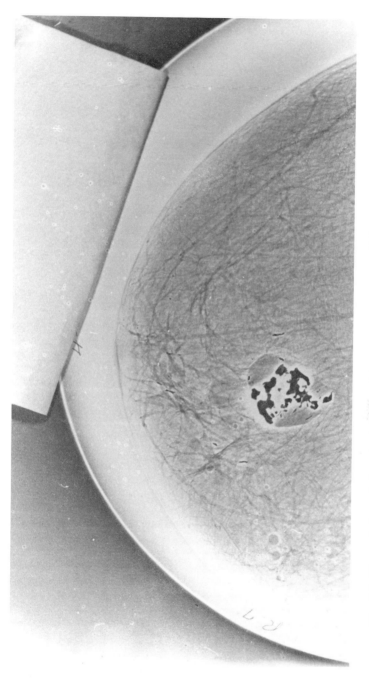

Fig. 3.4. The cephalocaudad projection of a right breast containing a 2.5-to-3-cm-in-dimension, palpable, rock-hard mass clinically suspicious for carcinoma. This has the classical radiographic appearance of a benign, partially calcified, degenerated fibroadenoma. The large conglomerate calcification is characteristic. There are also a few very small benign-appearing nodules medially and some benign linear ductal calcifications.

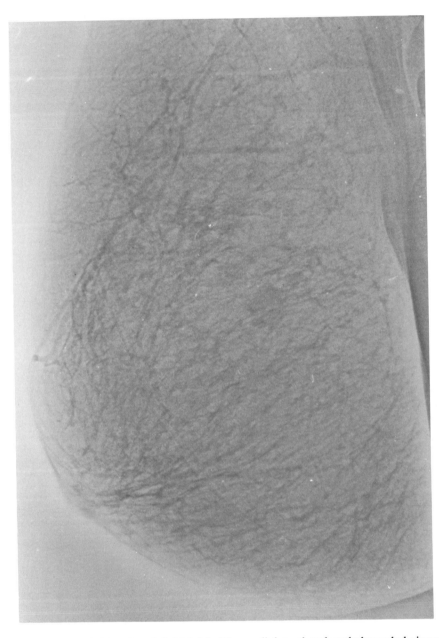

Figs. 3.5 (above) and 3.6 (right). The mediolateral and cephalocaudad views of a 1-cm-in-dimension slightly irregular mass without evident calcifications. The margins are not sharply demarcated, and the lesion should be regarded with suspicion and biopsied. This proved to be an infiltrating ductal carcinoma with negative axillary lymph nodes. The lesion was clinically occult.

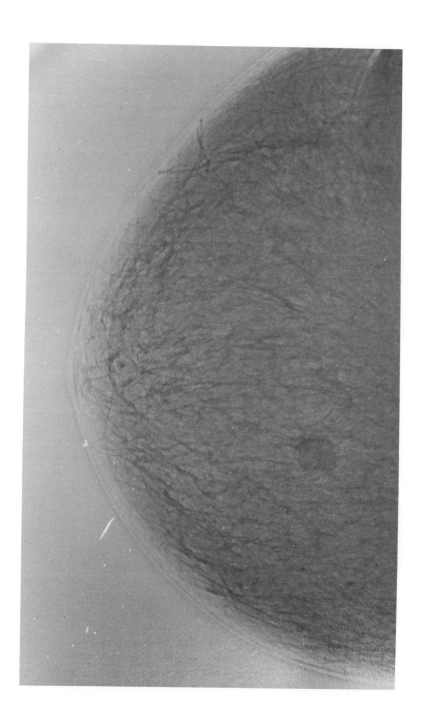

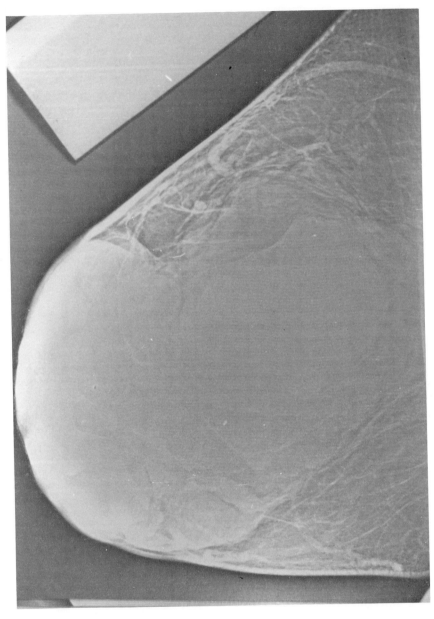

Figs. 3.7 (above) and 3.8 (right). Fig. 3.7 is a mediolateral view and Fig. 3.8 is a cephalocaudad view of the same breast with a very large multilobulated mass occupying almost two thirds of the entire breast in a young adult. There is no calcification. This is a giant fibroadenoma or cystosarcoma phylloides.

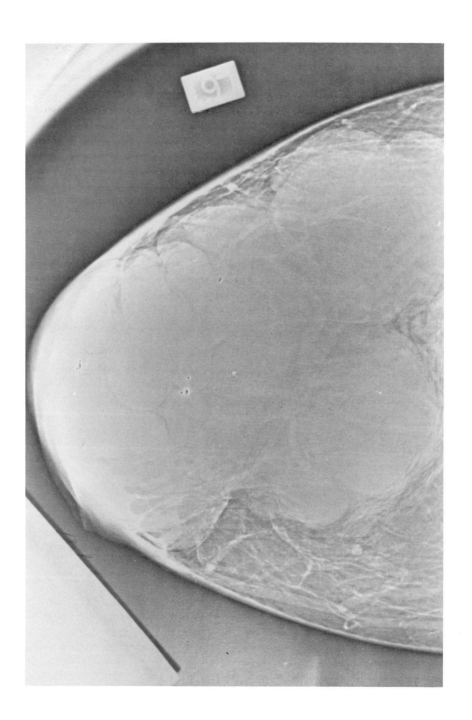

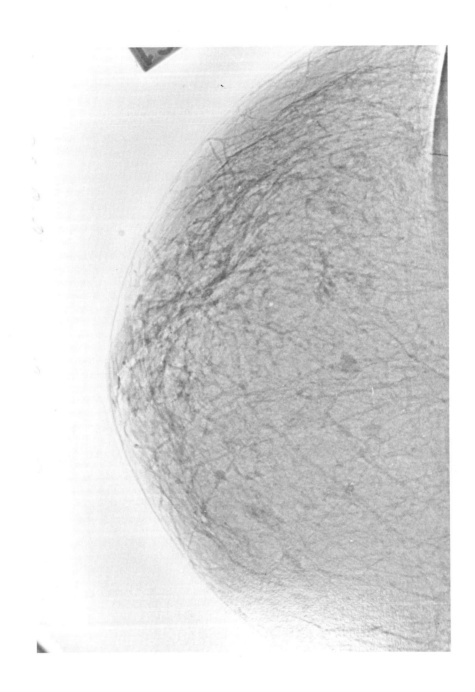

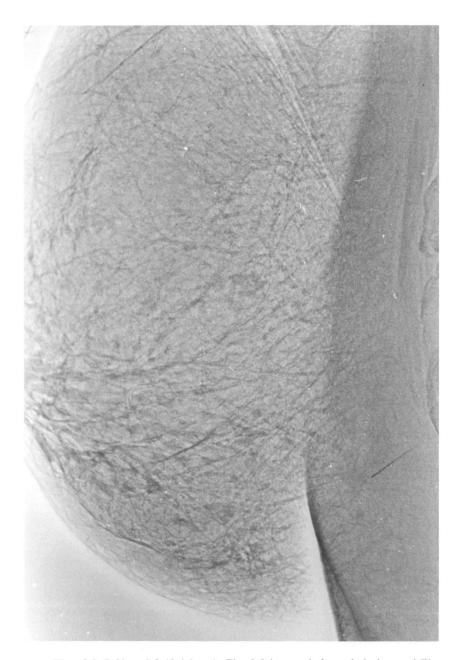

Figs. 3.9 (left) and 3.10 (above). Fig. 3.9 is a cephalocaudad view and Fig. 3.10 is a close-up of a portion of a lateral view showing a less-than-1-cm-in-dimension stellate mass in the lower outer quadrant of the left breast next to the chest wall. This is an infiltrating ductal and tubular carcinoma. The axillary lymph nodes were negative. The lesion was clinically occult. The visualization of the lesion on the lateral view is facilitated by the latitude of the Xerox process. The lesion is actually partially obscured by an overlying skin fold; however, the lesion is still quite discernible.

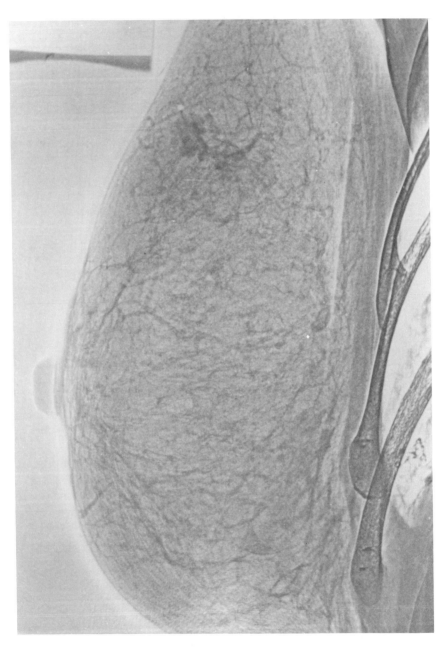

Figs. 3.11 (above) and 3.12 (right). Fig. 3.11 is a mediolateral view and Fig. 3.12 is the cephalocaudad projection of a 1-cm-in-dimension, clinically occult, irregular "knobby" mass in the upper outer quadrant of the left breast. This did not contain any evidence of calcification and was an infiltrating lobular carcinoma.

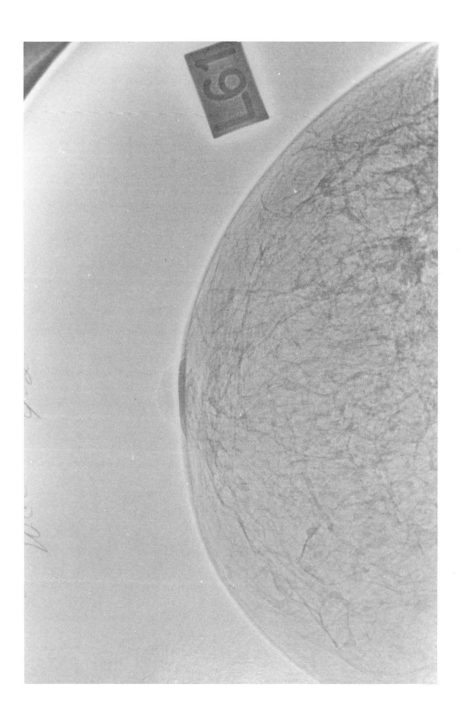

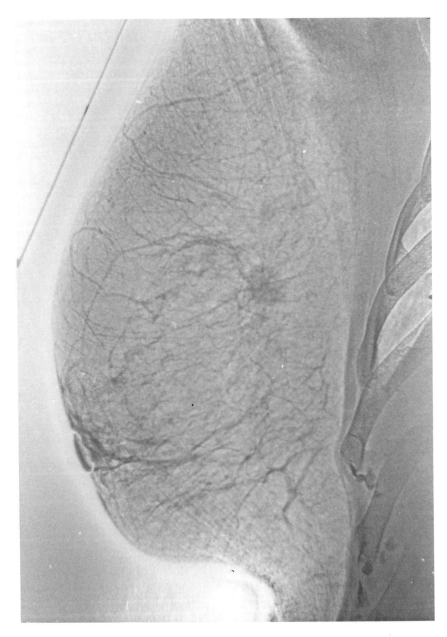

Figs. 3.13 (above) and 3.14 (right). Fig. 3.13 is a mediolateral projection and Fig. 3.14 is a cephalocaudad view of the same breast showing a 1-cm-in-dimension uncalcified mass in the upper outer quadrant. The margins of the mass are irregular and slightly stellate. There is a thickened ductlike structure extending upward anteriorly and medially from the mass. This was an infiltrating ductal carcinoma with negative axillary lymph nodes.

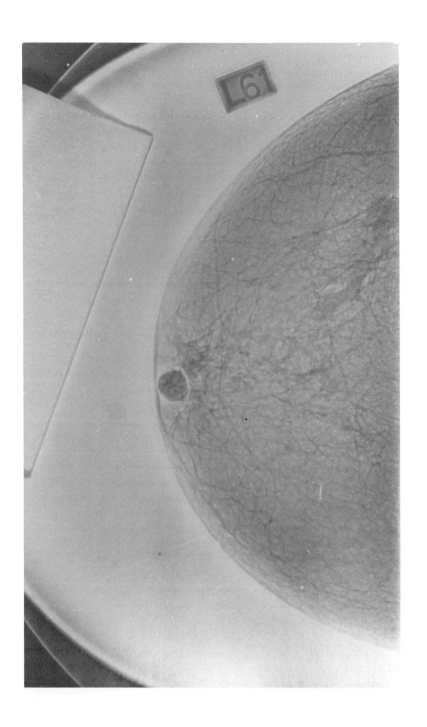

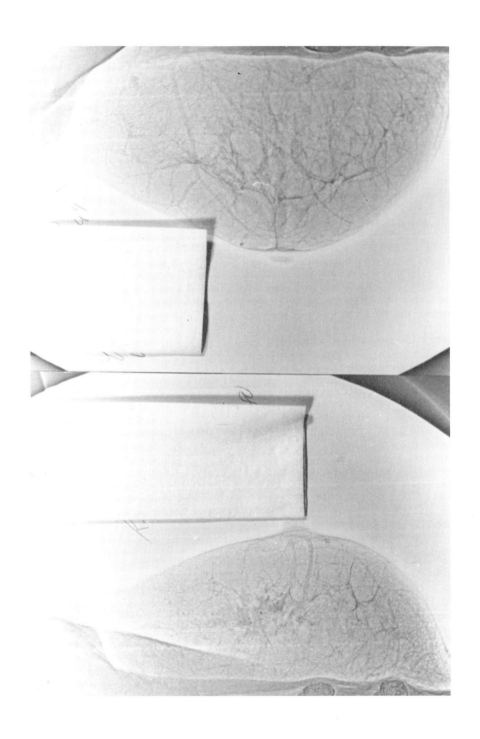

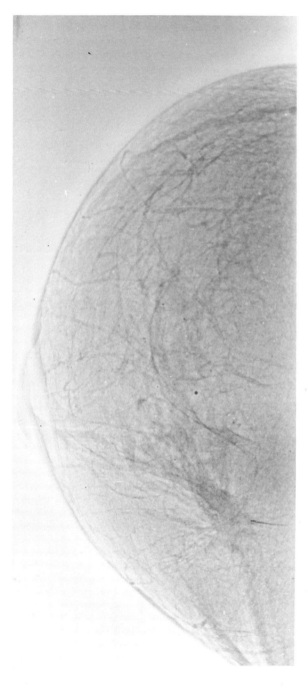

Figs. 3.15 (left) and 3.16 (above). Mediolateral views of each breast and cephalocaudad projection of the right breast. On the lateral views there is rather nonspecific increased density in the upper portion of the right breast. This illustrates how important it is to compare one side with the other. The density on the right breast is slightly suspicious, but since the other breast shows no similar density, it becomes much more suspicious. The cephalocaudad was also quite helpful because there is an obvious masslike density in this projection, as compared with the rather nonspecific density in the lateral view. The overlying skin thickening nearest the lesion in cephalocaudad projection was due to a previous biopsy scar. The lesion was an 0.8 cm infiltrating ductal carcinoma. The patient's axillary lymph nodes were negative. The lesion was clinically occult.

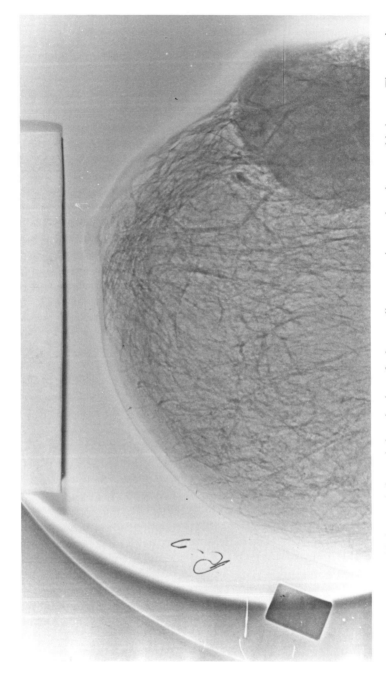

Fig. 3.17. This is a cephalocaudad projection of a large solitary mass in an otherwise atrophic breast. The mass is well circumscribed and has a fairly distinct margin. The mass is bulging the skin medially. This was a large, well-circumscribed infiltrating ductal carcinoma.

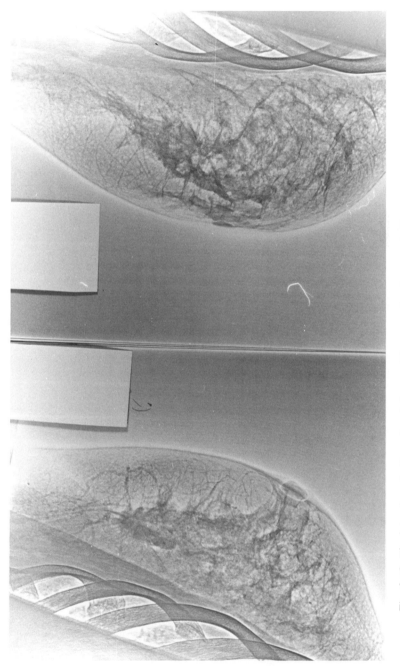

Fig. 3.18. The lateral projection of each breast. There are simultaneous infiltrating ductal carcinomas in the upper portion of each breast. There is a definite lobulated mass in the upper portion of the right breast (the picture on the **left**). There is a rather nonspecific increased density in the upper portion of the left breast (the picture on the **right**). There is slight nipple retraction on the left.

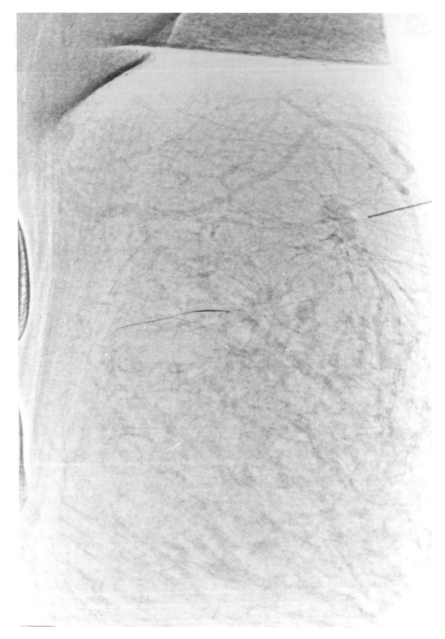

Fig. 3.19. A close-up magnified view of the superior portion of the lateral projection of the right breast. There are two very small, clinically occult primary infiltrating carcinomas. Note the adjacent increased vascular pattern.

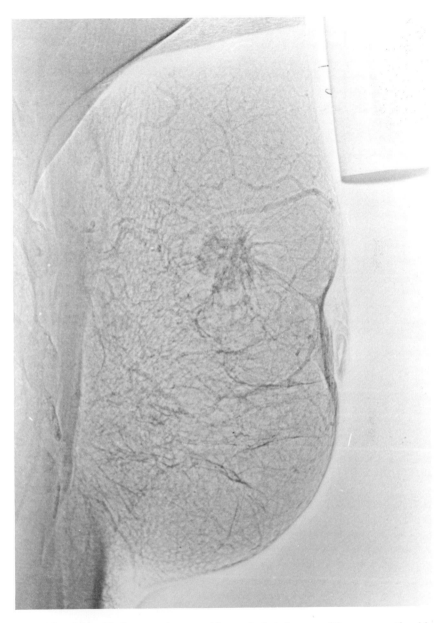

Fig. 3.20. Obvious carcinoma with a spiculated mass with a very noticeable area of skin thickening, skin retraction, and nipple retraction.

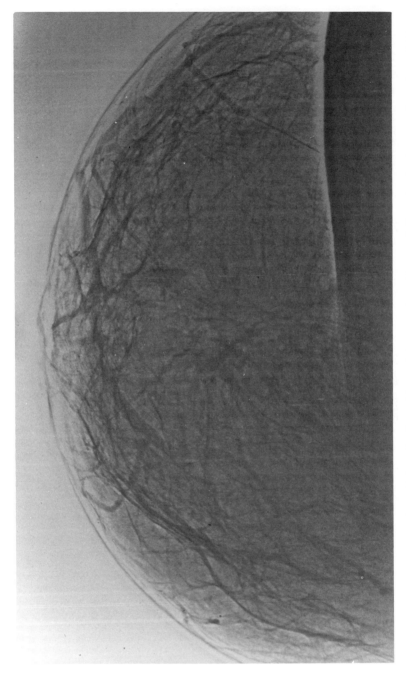

Fig. 3.21. A cephalocaudad projection with a subtle area of architectural distortion in the central portion of this view. A definite mass is not evident. No calcifications are seen. This is a very early subtle change due to the desmoplastic reaction by early scirrhous carcinoma. Note the prominent vein transversely across the breast anteriorly.

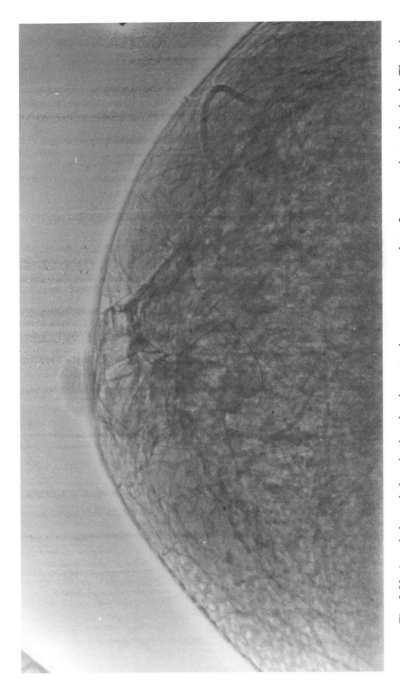

Fig. 3.22. A cephalocaudad projection showing a star-burst appearance about 2 cm posterior to the ripple. There is a very small associated mass. No calcifications are seen in the lesion. This is an early minimal infiltrating ductal carcinoma. Processing artifacts are on the image.

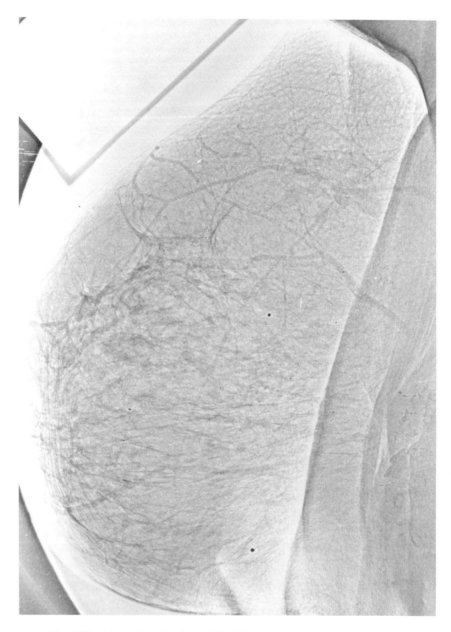

Fig. 3.23. A lateral projection of the left breast with a rather nonspecific area of increased density toward the axilla. A definite mass was not palpated in this area on physical examination; however, there was some rather nonspecific thickening detected. This was an infiltrating ductal carcinoma.

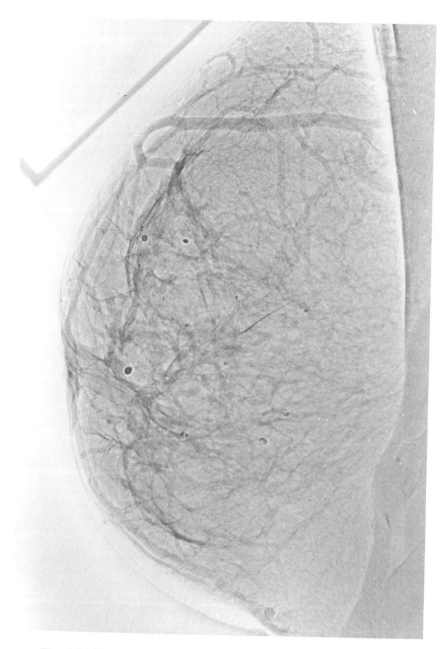

Figs. 3.24 (above) and 3.25 (following page). Lateral and cephalocaudad views, respectively, of a left breast with a 1-cm-in-dimension stellate mass in the central portion. The mass is more evident on the cephalocaudad view than on the lateral. There are several benign-appearing calcifications throughout the remainder of the breast. The venous pattern of the breast is exaggerated. This was a 1-cm-in-dimension infiltrating ductal carcinoma with negative lymph nodes. The lesion was clinically occult.

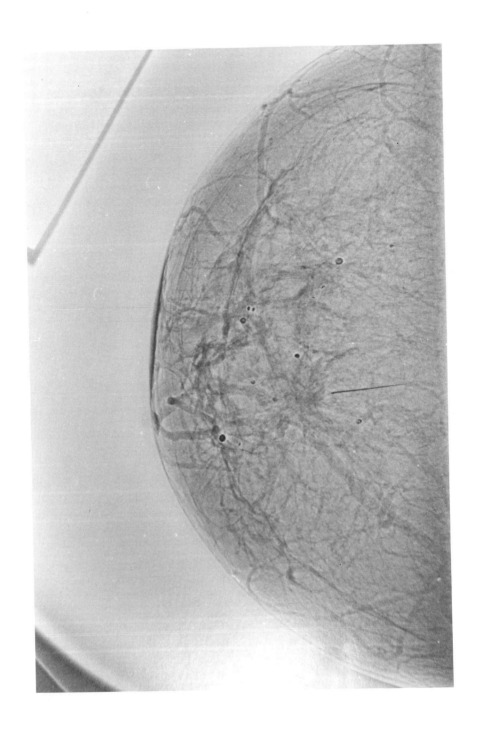

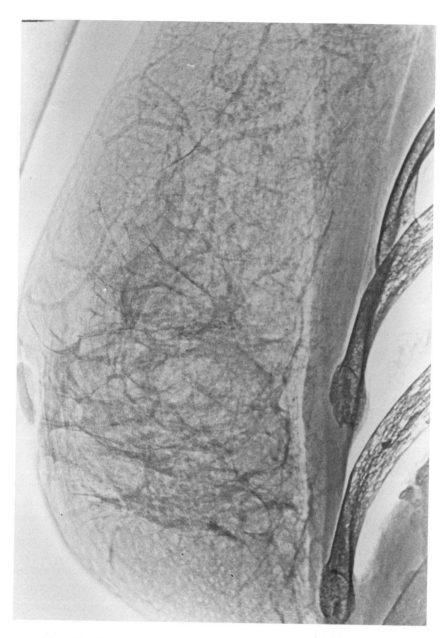

Figs. 3.26 (above) and 3.27 (following page). Lateral and cephalocaudad projections, respectively, of a small area of architectural distortion in the upper outer quadrant of the left breast. This is associated with a very few small punctate calcifications in the central portion of the lesion. There is skin thickening anteriorly in the lateral portion of the caudal view due to a previous biopsy site. The lesion was a very small infiltrating ductal carcinoma. Of eighteen axillary lymph nodes one was positive for metastatic disease.

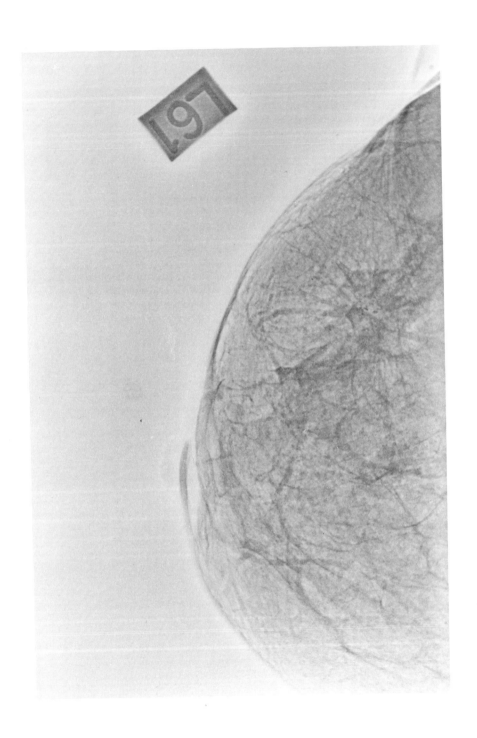

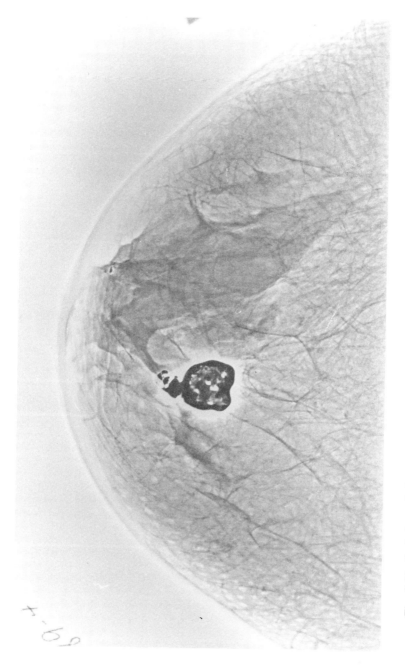

Fig. 3.28. Cephalocaudad projection of a 1.5-cm-in-dimension, degenerated, fibroadenoma with a large rock-hard calcification evident in the central portion of the breast.

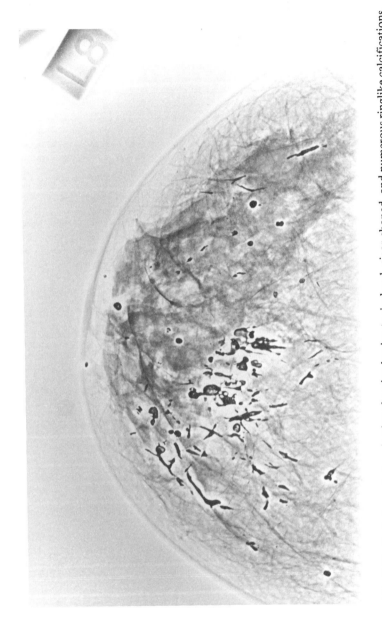

Fig. 3.29. Cephalocaudad projection showing benign typical rod, cigar-shaped, and numerous ringlike calcifications due to old so-called secretory disease.

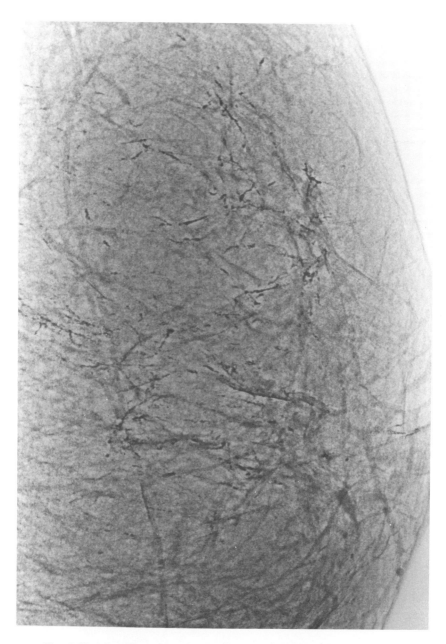

Fig. 3.30. Magnified view of a portion of a lateral image showing extensive ductal calcification, both of the linear and punctate variety. Some of the punctate calcifications are arranged in a linear fashion radiating toward the nipple as if they were distributed in the ducts. This is due to extensive comedocarcinoma. Compare this type of calcification with benign calcification in Fig. 3.29. The linear calcifications here are much finer than in the previous figure.

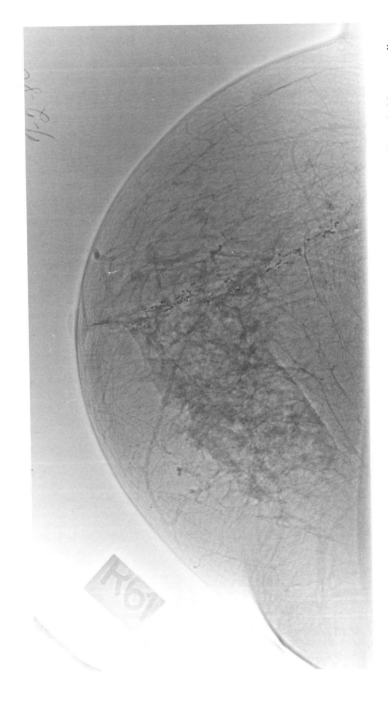

Fig. 3.31. Cephalocaudad projection revealing numerous punctate calcifications arranged in linear fashion extending from the subareolar region posteriorly almost to the chest wall. These were in an extensive carcinoma in situ.

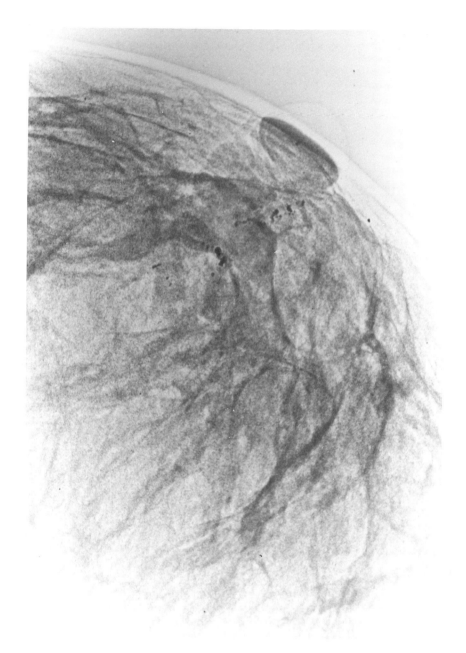

Fig. 3.32. Close-up projection of the subareolar region showing a small, fairly round mass immediately beneath the nipple with some adjacent punctate calcification arranged in a linear-type cluster. This was an infiltrating ductal carcinoma.

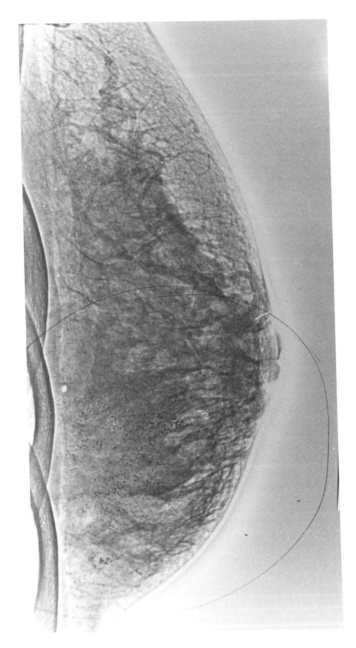

Figs. 3.33 (above) and 3.34 (right). Very large extensive diffuse carcinoma involving the entire lower half of the right breast. Fig. 3.33 is the lateral projection. Fig. 3.34 is a close-up magnified view of the cephalocaudad view showing the extensive punctate calcification in this extensive diffuse infiltrating ductal carcinoma.

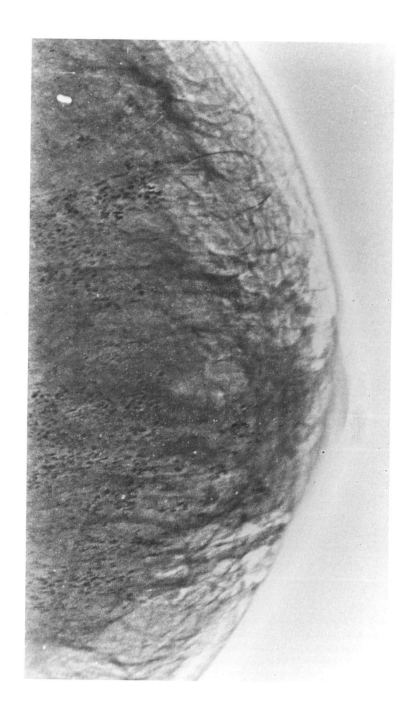

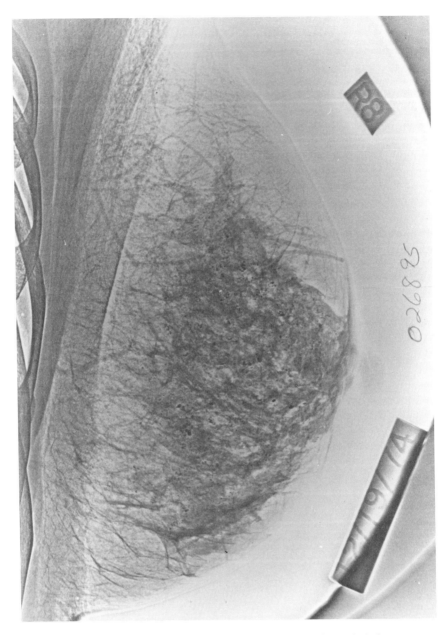

Figs. 3.35 (above) and 3.36 (right). Lateral and cephalocaudad views, respectively, of extensive diffuse punctate calcifications scattered throughout the entire breast. These have a somewhat similar appearance to the large carcinoma in Figs. 3.33. and 3.34. This is, however, due to benign sclerosing adenosis with diffuse calcifications throughout. It is very difficult to differentiate from the preceding case of extensive diffuse carcinoma shown in Figs. 3.33. and 3.34. It would almost be impossible to rule out at least some of these calcifications as being evidence of malignant disease.

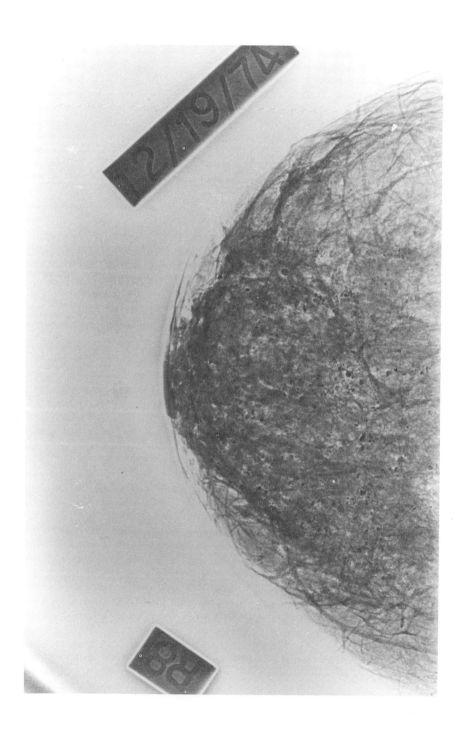

53

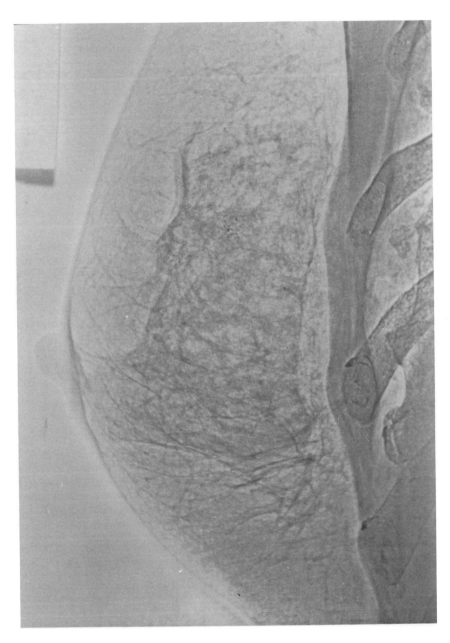

Fig. 3.37. There are two very small clusters of punctate calcification in the superior portion of this lateral projection. It is radiographically indeterminate in this type of situation whether the calcifications are symptomatic of benign or malignant disease, and biopsy is warranted.

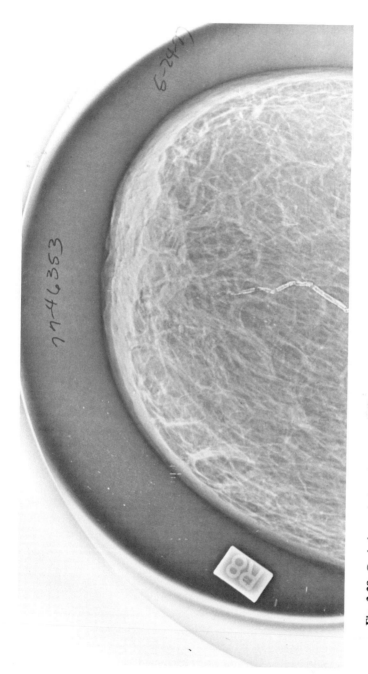

Fig. 3.38. Cephalocaudad projection showing extensive skin thickening of the entire breast. There is no underlying mass or distortion. There are a few scattered punctate calcifications in the central portion of the breast. Inflammatory carcinoma could produce this appearance; however, the changes are not specifically diagnostic. Inflammatory mastitis could produce similar changes, as could any other pathologic process causing diffuse skin thickening. This is a case of anasarca due to congestive heart failure.

punctate calcifications that renders them suspicious of being in malignant tissue. (Rarely, in a diffuse carcinoma or in a comedocarcinoma the calcification may be diffusely scattered throughout a large segment of the breast.) Benign calcifications are typically larger than malignant calcifications (Figs. 3.30, 3.33, and 3.34). As noted previously, some benign fibroadenomas, if they degenerate, will calcify with a characteristic popcorn-type calcification (Figs. 3.4 and 3.28). When this popcorn-type calcification is fully developed, it causes no problem in the differential diagnosis with malignant calcifications. Very rarely, however, as a degenerated fibroadenoma begins to calcify, it may produce a few small calcifications that are very difficult to distinguish from malignant calcifications. Large rod-shaped calcifications occur in the ducts on occasion (Fig. 3.29). They may range from a few millimeters to over a centimeter in length and from 1 to 3 cm in width. These rod- or cigar-shaped calcifications are readily recognized as benign disease calcifications. Doughnut- or ring-shaped calcifications are frequent and are ductal in origin and typically benign. They usually range in size from 1 to 3 mm in diameter.

Punctate calcifications can occur in either benign or malignant disease. Mammary dysplasia (the entire spectrum of fibrocystic disease) frequently causes punctate calcification either scattered or clustered. When scattered diffusely throughout the breast parenchyma, which is usually increased in density, the diagnosis of sclerosing adenosis is most likely (Figs. 3.35 and 3.36). Unfortunately, sclerosing adenosis can occur in localized form, causing some increased density, masses, and architectural distortion associated with clustered punctate calcifications that are radiographically indistinguishable from changes caused by malignant lesions.

Malignant calcifications are typically small punctate calcifications, either of the pinpoint dot variety or the size and shape of thin grains of sand. Sometimes they are branched (V-shaped or L-shaped branches, much like a breast duct would appear to branch). When the punctate calcifications are grouped in a cluster, they become quite suspicious. The clustered punctate calcifications may occur alone without any breast mass, architectural distortion, or abnormality in density being evident. This type of clustered punctate calcification cannot be differentiated radiographically into benign or malignant varieties and must have a biopsy for histologic diagnosis (Fig. 3.37). The clustered calcifications can also occur in a mass, leading to a more definitive radiographic diagnosis. Occasionally, the calcification may be adjacent to a mass in the ducts near the suspicious lesion, instead of actually being within the mass itself. The calcifications may vary from just a few—such as four to six punctate calcifications occurring within a 1 cm diameter area—to a more densely calcified cluster containing numerous punctate densities.

At times the calcifications of a suspicious nature are arranged in a linear fashion, as if in a duct, and occur in a radial fashion from the nipple or posterior areolar region to the posterior aspect of the breast (Figs. 3.31 and 3.32). This arrangement of calcification can also occur in either benign or malignant disease. To be considered in the differential diagnosis of such linearly arranged punctate calcifications are intraductal epithelial hyperplasia, papillomatosis, carcinoma in situ, comedocarcinoma, and infiltrating ductal carcinoma.

Mammary dysplasia, and especially sclerosing adenosis with punctate calcifications, are often very difficult to distinguish from a malignant process. Occasionally, fat necrosis will produce calcifications that also cause a diagnostic dilemma, and biopsy scars can produce similar appearances that can be indistinguishable from early carcinoma.

Rarely, the skin may be the site of scattered punctate calcifications, although these usually do not cause any problem in the differential diagnosis of breast parenchymal calcifications. If this confusion arises, different views of the breast may be obtained in differing degrees of obliquity to try to prove that the calcifications are indeed in the skin and not the breast parenchyma.

Architectural Distortion

Architectural distortion is often a subtle sign that is difficult for the novice to appreciate. It is difficult to describe precisely but has been described as areas of abnormal linear densities with small, radiating lines that liken to a pinwheel, spokewheel, or star-burst appearance (Fig. 3.21). This is caused at times by the retraction or scarring of benign breast connective tissue and also is caused by the desmoplastic reaction incited by early scirrhous carcinoma. It is not specific for malignancy since many benign processes can also produce distortion in the architectural pattern. Benign processes such as sclerosing adenosis, and especially scars from previous breast biopsies, can produce architectural distortion, and are indistinguishable from that produced by early scirrhous cancer. This is frequently a sign that will be evident before any mass or calcification has had time to develop in an early cancer and is, therefore, an important sign to be noted on the mammogram. This is also why it is so important to obtain a good history and physical examination, noting the site of any previous biopsies that could produce this architectural distortion and cause confusion in the differential diagnosis. Any time the normal breast connective tissue seems to be straightened or assumes anything other than its normal curvilinear symmetrical pattern, suspicion should be aroused. If small short lines develop that seem to run askew of the normal curvilinear stromal connective tissue, they are suspicious. If enough of these radiating lines become apparent and the typical starburst or spokewheel pattern is produced, with time a small mass may develop (Fig. 3.22). If calcifications become associated, the diagnosis is then fairly well established. However, as previously noted, benign disease, especially sclerosing adenosis and biopsy scars, can produce similar radiographic changes similar to those produced by early scirrhous carcinoma.

Nonspecific Areas of Increased Density

As previously mentioned, it is important to view the Xerox image of the breast side by side to its mate since they should be mirror images of each other. Any density that occurs in one breast that is not apparent in the similar location of its opposite mate should be regarded with some suspicion (Fig. 3.23). Again, the changes are not classical for malignancy since benign disease may produce similar areas of nonspecific increased density. This radiographic sign may be quite subtle at times.

Dilated Ducts

With the exception of the subareolar and lactiferous collecting ducts, the individual ducts of the breast are not normally seen on the mammogram. Occasionally, a solitary, very prominent ductlike structure will be evident, which should be considered suspicious. Occasionally, instead of a single dilated duct, a group of dilated ducts or an asymmetrical collection of ducts may be apparent. These abnormal ductlike structures may or may not contain calcifications, which may be either benign- or malignant-type calcifications. These abnormal ductlike structures can be due to benign diseases such as benign ductal epithelial hyperplasia, ductal ectasia, secretory disease (in which the ducts become dilated and filled with epithelial debris that may or may not calcify, with large benign rodlike calcifications), and papillomatosis. Occasionally, benign doughnut- or ringlike calcifications may occur. Plasma cell mastitis may produce a subareolar density, occasionally with some dilated ductlike structures extending posteriorly from an otherwise homogeneous subareolar masslike density. In malignancy the ducts may become dilated adjacent to an obvious carcinoma, (Figs. 3.13 and 3.14) but may dilate without an evident associated adjacent mass. Carcinoma in situ, comedocarcinoma, or early invasive carcinoma may dilate ducts and may or may not be associated with punctate calcifications arranged in a linear fashion within the dilated ductlike structure. A dilated duct or asymmetrical group of dilated ducts is not a frequent sign of cancer, and the changes can be quite subtle, especially if they occur in a dysplastic breast or one with a so-called prominent ductal pattern. However, when a dilated ductlike structure is prominent — and especially if it contains punctate calcifications arranged in a linear fashion — the changes are quite suspicious for carcinoma.

Developing Densities

Any density previously not evident that develops on subsequent mammograms should be regarded as suspicious. This is true especially in a postmenopausal breast that should be undergoing atrophy. Only when a previous mammogram is available for comparison is it possible to recognize this sign. This can be a very valuable sign, however, in recognizing a carcinoma that is beginning to develop. Not all developing densities or masses will be malignant, even in the postmenopausal age group. Even benign masses may rarely appear within the breasts of postmenopausal age, and rarely a postmenopausal benign mass may enlarge. These are suspicious and most should be biopsied. Metastatic nodules may also appear in the breast as developing densities and are frequently multiple and may even be bilateral. They can appear as fairly well circumscribed nodules and have a benign appearance or may be more classically malignant in appearance, with irregular, knobby margins. Also to be noted is any change in the character of the margin of what was originally presumed to be a benign nodule or mass. This should be regarded as suspicious, especially when the previously well demarcated margin changes to an indistinct margin or becomes knobby, irregular, or stellate in appearance. A very slow-growing lesion that was originally presumed to be a tiny benign nodule may take a year or longer to show some growth on the X ray and to change in marginal characteristics and thus becomes a more suspicious lesion. The doubling time of breast cancer has been calculated to range from 23 to 209 days [Donegan and Spratt 1979].

In addition to the above primary signs of suspicion, there are some secondary signs that must also be noted in interpreting mammograms. These are nonspecific in nature but should arouse some suspicion when noted and add to the degree of suspiciousness when associated with some of the aforementioned primary signs of carcinoma. These are enlarged, solid axillary lymph nodes; increased vascularity, either localized or generalized; skin thickening, either localized or generalized; skin retraction; or nipple retraction. Some posteriorly located lesions may cause obliteration of the retromammary space on the lateral view. This implies fixation to the chest wall.

MANAGEMENT

When a suspicious lesion or area that is clinically occult is noted on the mammogram, and biopsy is deemed necessary, the lesion is localized and diagrammed for the surgeon. Measurements are made on the mammogram in relation to the vertical and transverse nipple lines. The depth posterior to the nipple or from the chest wall anteriorly and the depth from the skin are measured. The lesion is then plotted on a diagram of the breast and described so that the surgeon and the pathologist know not only where the area of suspicion is located but also what the radiographic nature of the lesion is — whether it is a mass, an architectural distortion, a calcification, etcetera. It is a very difficult surgical task to biopsy some of these lesions, which are at times almost microscopic in size. It should be realized that some of these small lesions appear to change somewhat in location from where they appear to be on X rays. The X-ray images are made with compression and with the patient in a recumbent lateral position for the mediolateral projection, with the patient sitting upright, for a cephalocaudad view. When the patient assumes a supine position on the operating room table, the apparent location of a very small lesion, especially in a large, pendulous, lax breast, may change somewhat in position as compared with the apparent position on the mammograms.

An ample biopsy specimen must be obtained, and most of the time X rays of the specimen — so-called specimen mammograms — are obtained by the pathologist to see if the area of concern has been excised. If the area of concern is not evident in the specimen mammogram, the surgeon is immediately informed and a larger biopsy specimen is obtained. The specimen mammogram allows the pathologist to identify the lesion rapidly and localize the area to make histologic sections. In very small lesions most pathologists prefer not to prepare frozen sections but to preserve all of the tissue for permanent sectioning. In larger, gross lesions, obtaining frozen sections, at times, is an acceptable procedure.

Good communication and teamwork among the referring physician, radiologist, pathologist, and the surgeon will enable more of these minimal cancers to be detected, properly biopsied, diagnosed, and managed accordingly. The clinician should inform the radiologist as to whether there are clinical symptoms or signs; the radiologist must inform the pathologist and surgeon of the location and characteristics of the area of concern; and the pathologist must inform the surgeon as to whether that area has, indeed, been excised. This communication facilitates proper patient management in detecting, excising, and confirming minimal cancers.

REFERENCES

Donegan WL, and Spratt JS (1979) Cancer of the breast, 2nd ed. Philadelphia, W. B. Saunders.

Egan RL (ed) (1976) Technologist's guide to detection of early breast cancer by mammography, thermography and xeroradiography. Chicago, Ill., American College of Radiology.

Wolfe, JN (1972) Xeroradiography of the breast. Springfield, Ill., Charles C. Thomas.

4

Clinical Examination
and Thermography

Ned D. Rodes
Dinah K. Pearson

CLINICAL EXAMINATION PROCESS

When the Breast Cancer Detection Demonstration Project (BCDDP) contract began in Columbia, Missouri, on June 1, 1974, one registered nurse was employed to do the breast palpations. The medical director of the program, a surgeon, trained this nurse to do thorough breast examinations. The training included lectures on anatomy and physiology, followed by a lengthy internship.

The medical director personally examined each of the participants for several weeks. The nurse was present as he examined the participant and explained the examination process and his observations to her. The nurse then reexamined the woman in order to replicate the findings.

As the nurse's skill and confidence increased, she began to perform the initial examination with the medical director present to reexamine and confirm her interpretation. After a period of several weeks, the nurse clinician assumed the responsibility for performing the examinations, but the medical director was readily available for consultation on difficult or abnormal findings.

Unlike the radiologists who did not know the woman's name or have access to any of her medical history information at the time of interpretation, the nurse had the medical history available. After spending a few minutes establishing rapport with the participant, the nurse was able to obtain additional information about family history of breast cancer, parity, breast feeding, hormone therapy, performance of self-breast examination, previous breast surgery, date of the last menstral period, time of the last examination by a physician, and any present breast complaints as well as details of past breast disease history.

The physical inspection and palpation of the breasts included having the participant place her hands on her hips while seated on the examination table. The nurse asked the participant to press her hands firmly down and flex her chest muscles and then to elevate her arms over her head. The examiner visually inspected the breasts for symmetry of shape, size, and contour and also checked the nipples and skin surfaces for any abnormalities.

Next, the participant was placed in a supine position. The participant's arm was placed above her head on the side to be examined. With her fingers flat and by using the fingertips of all four fingers on both hands, the nurse firmly palpated the breast tissue in a clockwise motion. The palpation began at the outermost portion of the breast at the 12 o'clock position. The examination progressed in continuous circles in toward and including the nipple. Finally, the nipple was gently milked to check for any discharge. If an abnormal discharge was found, a pap smear was obtained. The axillary and supraclavicular regions were also examined for evidence of bulging, edema, discoloration, or retraction.

If a mass or thickening was palpated, the nurse carefully measured it and also described its texture, mobility, and shape. Finally, she diagramed the area on the standard form (see Appendix A).

Some bias may have been introduced on recall examinations because the nurse would know that the woman had returned prior to her routine annual visit because of a possible abnormality. Occasionally, one of the radiologists would send written instructions to the nurse to examine a particular area of the breast for a biopsy scar, mole, or possible abnormality.

As the nurse examined the participant, she explained her findings while teaching each woman individually to examine her own breasts. The woman had already viewed a seven-minute film from the American Cancer Society (ACS) entitled "How to Examine Your Breasts." This provided the woman with the basic information necessary. The time with the nurse provided her with an opportunity to ask the nurse questions while practicing breast self-examination (BSE).

The nurse carefully demonstrated areas that she felt might be of concern to the woman, such as the firm ridge of tissue along the lower portion of the breast, which is common especially in women with large breasts. Other noted areas included thickenings, areas of nodularity, cysts, or other masses. These areas were particularly important when the woman was referred to her private physician.

At the conclusion of her examination and BSE-training session, the nurse gave the participant a pamphlet—also entitled "How to Examine Your Breasts"—that was provided by the ACS to accompany the film on BSE. The woman was instructed to examine her breasts each month, one week following the onset of menses. If she was postmenopausal, the day of the month was not important, but monthly BSE was still recommended.

The participants were advised to contact their physician if any abnormalities were detected prior to their scheduled annual BCDDP appointment.

On her initial visit the participant spent approximately 20 minutes with the nurse clinician. Subsequent screening visits were usually shorter but included the same type of physical inspection of the breasts by the nurse clinician as well as a review of BSE.

Following the first year of operation, a second full-time nurse clinician was employed to do half of the screening examinations, which increased from 5,000 to 10,000 per year. This nurse was trained by the medical director as well as by the first nurse clinician.

QUALITY CONTROL FOR CLINICAL EXAMINATION

In 1977 the National Cancer Institute required that each project institute a system of quality control procedures for the physical examination. Columbia BCDDP No. 25 attempted to comply with this requirement by employing two surgery residents to recheck a sample of the nurses' examinations. The residents were located next door at the state cancer hospital and came to the project on a random basis (as their schedules permitted). They were required to reexamine at least 10 percent of all the participants and record their findings.

This protocol was followed for a period of six months, at which time it was suspended pending review. Each participant in the sample was closely followed for a period of two years to determine how accurate the nurses and surgery residents had been in performing and evaluating the breast examinations. Each examiner was asked to interpret the examination as (1) normal; (2) breast abnormalities present, probably benign; or (3) breast abnormalities present, suspicious of malignancy.

During the six-month period more than 500 women were included in the quality control sample. The two-year follow-up of each case revealed that the nurses' evaluations had been essentially correct in every case.

THERMOGRAPHY

Thermography is a technique for measuring the infrared heat given off by the body. The BCDDPs were charged with determining the effectiveness of thermography as a tool for breast cancer screening.

At the Columbia project independence of examinations was given high priority. This was one of the reasons that a radiologist specially trained and experienced in thermography was employed to interpret the examinations. This radiologist did not have access to the participant's name, medical history information, or the mammography and physical findings at the time of interpretation.

A technician was trained by the radiologist in charge of thermography to obtain the images. In addition, the technician completed a week of training at the BCDDP in Oklahoma City. All three of the (mammographic) radiologic technologists were trained to fill in for the technician during breaks and absenses.

In preparation for the thermographic examination each woman was disrobed to the waist and placed for 8 to 10 minutes in a booth partitioned by curtains. The "cooling" room temperature was maintained between 68° and 70°F. While the woman was seated, she held on to a pole with each hand to keep her arms away from her body. During this time she watched the film entitled "How to Examine Your Breasts." The cooling process provided equilibration of the participant's skin temperature. After 10 minutes the woman stood at a distance of 24 inches in front of the thermography machine with her arms raised over her head.

The thermographic machine was a Spectrotherm 1000 made by General Electric. A Polaroid camera was attached to the machine, and Polaroid coatless black and white film was used to record a minimum of four images for each participant.

Each photograph was accompanied by temperature lines that allowed the radiologist to compare the relative temperatures of the two breasts. In three of the four standard views the background was white, so these were known as black-hot views since dark areas were areas of heat. On these views the thermographic technician placed the temperature line through what she determined visually to be the hottest area of either breast. These three views were anterior-posterior and oblique views from the right and left.

The fourth standard view was a white-hot anterior-posterior view (Fig. 4.1). On this fourth picture the technician attempted to place the temperature line through the two areolae. In many cases, the women were not symmetric enough to place the horizontal line through both areolae.

The four Polaroid pictures were mounted on one 8½" × 11" cardboard sheet and then attached to the standard data form (see Appendix A). The radiologist interpreted each set of films, comparing the background temperatures of the two breasts, the symmetry of the vascular patterns for number, vessel width, and temperature, and the overall temperature levels of the two areolae. This information, along with the interpretation of the examination, was recorded on the form by the radiologist.

Examples of several types of abnormalities detected are shown in Figs. 4.2 through 4.6.

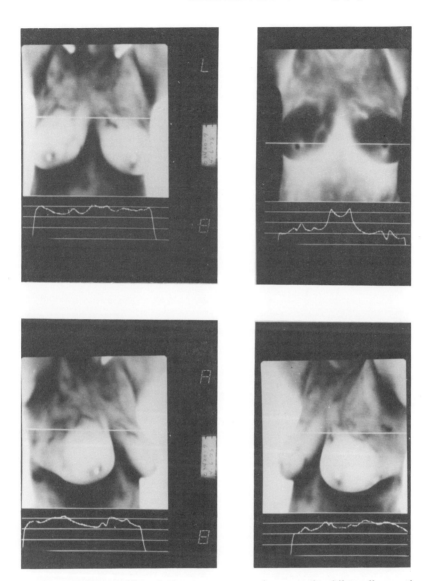

Fig. 4.1. This participant's thermograms were interpreted as bilaterally negative on each of four sets of annual examinations. She has almost avascular breasts. No abnormality was detected on either mammography or clinical palpation during five years of participation in the BCDDP. (Thermography was discontinued by the National Cancer Institute prior to her fifth annual visit.)

On each set of thermograms the film in the **upper left** is the black-hot anterior-posterior view, the **upper right** is the white-hot anterior-posterior view, the **lower left** is the right oblique, and the **lower right** is the left oblique.

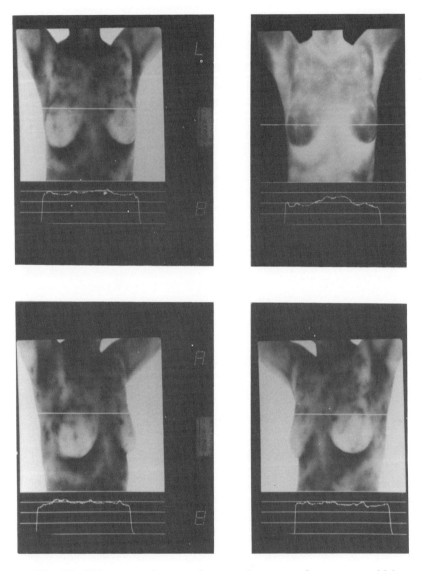

Fig. 4.2. This woman has a rather prominent vascular pattern, which was interpreted as normal on each of four annual visits. The mammograms and physical examinations were also unremarkable on each visit.

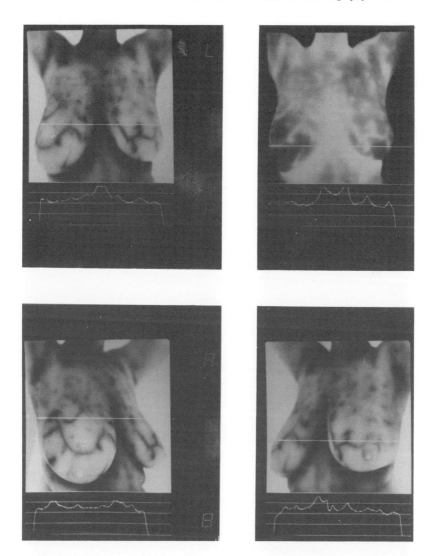

Fig. 4.3. This participant's thermograms were interpreted as asymmetric on her fourth annual visit. The radiologist indicated that she had diffuse areas of increased heat emission in the left breast. Furthermore, both the anteroposterior projection and oblique projection of the left breast showed increased heat emission, the background temperature of the two breasts was not symmetric, and there were an increased number of veins and an increased temperature of veins bilaterally.

On the same occasion a mass visualized on mammography led to a biopsy recommendation of the left breast. The biopsy was performed, and a fibroadenoma was excised from the 11 o'clock position of the left breast.

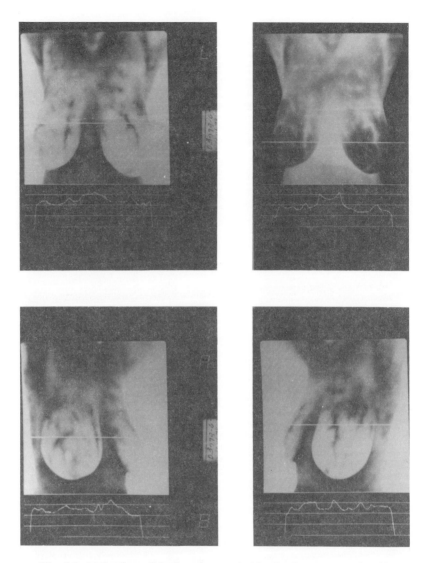

Fig. 4.4. At the time of the fourth annual visit, the thermograms for this participant were interpreted as bilaterally abnormal. The right breast had an increased number of veins in the lower inner quadrant. The left breast had an increased number of veins, an increased caliber of veins, and an increased temperature of veins in upper portion.

On the same occasion the nurse clinician described a biopsy scar in the lower portion of the left breast but detected no abnormalities. A biopsy was recommended on the basis of mammographic findings in the right breast. A 2.0 cm indeterminate mass was described on mammography in the 12 o'clock radial. The biopsy of this area found a small fibroadenoma as well as fibrocystic disease.

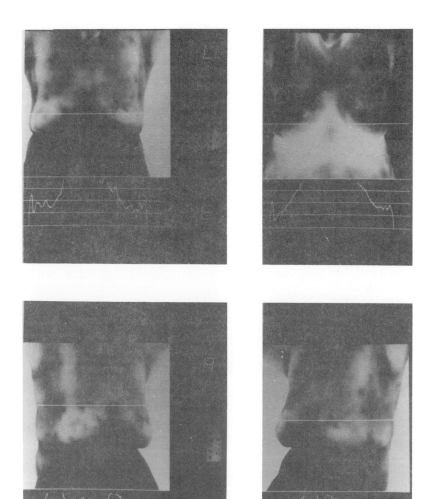

Fig. 4.5. The radiologist complained that this participant was very difficult to cool properly for the examination. It was suggested at the time of the second annual visit that supine cooling be considered for participants of this type in order to obtain a more satisfactory examination. However, in spite of this handicap the radiologist interpreted the examination to show an asymmetry of the vascular pattern in the lower inner quadrant of the left breast.

On this same occasion the nurse clinician described no areas of concern, but the mammograms revealed an area of concern in the upper outer portion of the left breast. The biopsy of this area confirmed the presence of a tubular adenocarcinoma. The woman had a modified radical mastectomy, and all 18 lymph nodes showed lymphoid hyperplasia.

The BCDDP has carefully followed this participant for six years, and to date she has not had any signs of recurrence.

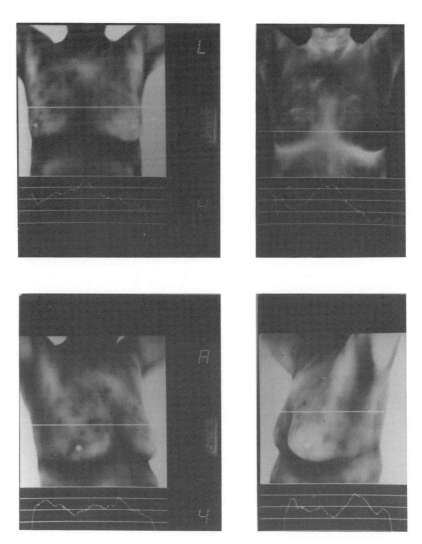

Fig. 4.6. At the time of her third annual visit, this participant's thermograms were interpreted as abnormal on the right. The background temperature was described as asymmetric. Diffuse areas of heat emission were noted in the right breast.

The vascular pattern of the two breasts was described as asymmetric and the distortion was in the upper inner, lower outer, and lower inner quadrants of the right breast (increased number and temperature of veins). The two areolae did not have an equal temperature, with increased heat noted in the right breast.

The nurse clinician did not describe any abnormalities on the third annual visit, but local areas of nonspecific increased density were described in the central portion of each breast on mammography. At the time of the weekly chart conference, the senior medical staff reviewed the case, and it was their combined judgment that a biopsy should be recommended in the right breast.

The pathologist who reviewed the tissue slides after the biopsy indicated that the final diagnosis was microductular-type infiltrating adenocarcinoma. The woman had a radical mastectomy, and all 21 lymph nodes were negative.

During five years of follow-up by the BCDDP this woman has had no indication of recurrence.

PART II

Modeling and Analysis

Some of the analytical techniques employed in this research project are fairly widely understood, while some are somewhat more esoteric. To provide the reader with background as needed, we begin this part with a chapter illustrating the less common techniques and describing a new contribution to decision analysis developed for this project. In subsequent chapters we evaluate screening accuracy at Breast Cancer Detection Demonstration Project (BCDDP) No. 25, present our results on breast cancer risk profiles, map out optimal and suboptimal screening protocols by risk level, and develop optimal mammographic examination schedules using a decision analytic model for risk-benefit evaluations.

5

Analytical Methods

John K. Gohagan
Edward L. Sptiznagel

Complex analytical studies such as ours typically require the use of a variety of quantitative techniques. The techniques we employed fall into three major classes: decision analysis, benefit-cost analysis, and mathematical statistics. Our analytical approach is generally like that of a decision analyst, an operations researcher, or a systems analyst.

Decision analysis provides the overall organizing paradigm for the study because the fundamental objective is to find in some sense "best" detection strategies for women with specific risk profiles. These strategies or decision alternatives are evaluated on a cost-benefit basis, benefits in this case taking the form of cost savings from early detection and avoidance of unnecessary tests and surgery. Some widely understood and some rather esoteric statistical techniques are used to summarize and extract basic information from our large data base, smooth data for input into decision analysis algorithms, and determine the groupings of both epidemiological and test outcome variables, that most accurately predict disease. Of necessity we invented a unique computerized decision analytic procedure that identifies, evaluates, and ranks all possible single- and multimodality diagnostic protocols. This algorithm represents an original contribution to the field of decision analysis and is applicable to medical and nonmedical problems alike.

The main avenues of our analysis and the techniques employed are outlined in Table 5.1. Our purpose in this chapter is to illustrate the more important of these methods using easily understood examples. In the limited space available we cannot hope to teach the reader any of the methods. But we want to provide some insight for the novice into the logic

TABLE 5.1.
Main Avenues of Analysis and Techniques Employed

Epidemiologic risk assessment
  Hypothesis testing for identifying statistically significant individual features
  Multivariate discriminate and regression analyses to find statistically significant
    discriminating feature groupings
Modality evaluation
  Cross-tabulation frequencies for preliminary evaluations of alternative modality
    interpretation rules
  Logistic regression to determine optimal groupings of examination facts for defining
    positive and negative outcomes for individual modalities
  Log-linear modeling of cross-classified data to estimate sensitivity and specificity
    for individual modalities and multimodality strategies
  Logistic regression to find optimal multimodality feature groupings
Strategy selection
  New strategy identification, evaluation, and ranking algorithm developed in the
    course of our research
  Basic principles of benefit-cost and decision analysis

Note: Noninferential statistical techniques like frequency distributions and summary
statistics are not listed.

of the various methods and to illustrate generally how they were applied in
this study.

DECISION ANALYSIS

Decision analysis is a methodology developed by statisticians, math-
ematicians, operations researchers, and economists for analyzing and comparing complex decision alternatives [Gohagan 1980]. Decision problems
are organized into decision alternatives with attendant costs and possible
impacts. Probabilistic links between actions and impacts are established
statistically or, where necessary, judgmentally. Decision objectives are
postulated. A decision-making perspective is adopted and changed as appropriate to develop deep insight into the problem. Initial analyses are completed and interpreted. And subsequent, usually extensive, sensitivity
analyses are conducted to determine wide ranges of conditions under which
specific decision alternatives are preferable.

Simple decision problems can be portrayed in tree form. For example,
if an asymptomatic woman not yet examined by any means had to choose
whether to have a mammogram, an abbreviated version of her decision problem could be diagrammed as in Fig. 5.1. The tree is highly simplified in that
it presumes unequivocal, meaningful definitions of positive and negative
mammograms, whereas we know that a wide variety of definitions are
possible; furthermore, experience suggests that in many situations

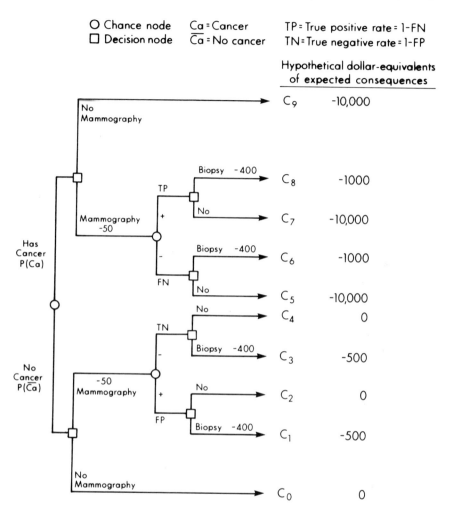

Fig. 5.1. Abbreviated version of mammography versus no-exam decision problem.

dichotomization itself may be inappropriate. Also the tips of the tree are truncated, thereby masking the wide array of possible impacts that could follow upon any sequence of test results and actions for cancerous or non-cancerous women. Although much more complex trees more accurately representing the decision problem can be drawn, this one is good enough for illustrative purposes, and such simple trees once computerized provide a basic structure that can be modified and evaluated with relative ease.

The probability $P(Ca)$ is the chance that the woman has cancer at the time of decision. This is a number one cannot know with precision. It must be estimated from preexamination information including incidence and prevalence data modified to reflect epidemiological risk features exhibited by the woman at the time of decision. The true positive rate (*TP*), the true negative rate (*TN*), or their complements *FN* and *FP*, respectively, are specific to individual mammographic practices and should be estimated from clinic-specific data.[1]

The expected consequences C_0 through C_9 are averages that must be estimated from usually complex probability distributions for consequences. These are not clinic-specific impacts but are to some degree individual-specific. They are the dollar-equivalent net values of any benefits of early detection less applicable procedural costs like mammography, biopsy, surgery, and adjuvant therapy plus opportunity costs like income foregone, psychological costs, and so forth.

Five possible decision strategies are incorporated into the tree. They are: do nothing for now; do mammography and biopsy only if positive; do mammography and biopsy only if negative; do mammography and biopsy regardless of the findings; and, finally, do mammography but do no biopsy under any circumstance (Table 5.2). But some of these are not viable. For example, it makes no sense to do mammography and not use the resulting information, for that increases costs to no advantage. Thus, the last two strategies are not viable. Neither does it make sense to recommend biopsy on the basis of a negative examination unless the false positive rate exceeds the true positive rate, which hopefully would never be the case unless positive and negative examinations were inappropriately defined.

The same strategies apply whether or not the woman in question actually has cancer, because her actual status is unknown. However, the relative worths of individual strategies vary according to the estimated preexamination probability $P(Ca)$ that cancer is present. Thus, one evaluates all viable strategies, first assuming that cancer is present and subsequently that it is not, and chooses a course of action on the basis of how the chance of cancer modifies these results. Strategies offering larger weighted net benefits to the woman are naturally preferred, and the strategy with the largest weighted net benefits is most desirable.

TABLE 5.2.
Possible Decision Strategies for Fig. 5.1

	Strategy Decision
S_1	Do nothing for now
Do mammography and	
S_2	Biopsy only if positive
S_3	Biopsy only if negative
S_4	Biopsy in either case
S_5	Biopsy in neither case

The evaluation and selection process is easily perceived by example. If one has determined that the true positive (*TP*) and false positive (*FP*) rates for the clinical practice are 70 percent and 20 percent, respectively, that the net of benefits and costs for detection, unnecessary biopsy, and missed cancers were 1,000, 500, and 10,000 dollar-equivalents, respectively, that mammography costs $50, and that biopsy costs $400, one would evaluate the strategies as shown in Table 5.3 using the following expressions:

$$\text{Expected Net Value } (S_i) = P(Ca) \begin{pmatrix} \text{Net Value of} \\ \text{Strategy } S_i \\ \text{to Women} \\ \text{with Cancer} \end{pmatrix}$$

$$+ P(\overline{Ca}) \begin{pmatrix} \text{Net Value of} \\ \text{Strategy } S_i \\ \text{to Women} \\ \text{without Cancer} \end{pmatrix}$$

$$\begin{matrix} \text{Net Value of} \\ \text{Strategy } S_i \\ \text{to Women} \\ \text{with Cancer} \end{matrix} = TP \begin{pmatrix} \text{Net Value} \\ \text{of Detection} \end{pmatrix} + FN \begin{pmatrix} \text{Net Value} \\ \text{of a Miss} \end{pmatrix}$$

$$+ \begin{matrix} \text{Cost of} \\ \text{Mammogram} \end{matrix}$$

$$\begin{matrix} \text{Net Value of} \\ \text{Strategy } S_i \\ \text{to Women} \\ \text{without Cancer} \end{matrix} = FP \begin{pmatrix} \text{Net Value} \\ \text{of Inappropriate} \\ \text{Surgery} \end{pmatrix} + TN \begin{pmatrix} \text{No} \\ \text{Costs} \end{pmatrix}$$

$$+ \begin{matrix} \text{Cost of} \\ \text{Mammogram} \end{matrix}$$

As indicated previously, strategy selection is sensitive to the preexamination probability of cancer, $P(Ca)$. When there is a 10 percent chance that a woman has cancer, strategy S_2, biopsy only on positive mammogram, is best. The second-best strategy in this circumstance is S_1, do nothing at this time. The cost differential for the two strategies is quite large at 660 dollar-equivalents, pointing to the much greater utility of S_2. However, when the chance of disease is 1 percent, the best strategy on the basis of the data provided in this example is S_1, postpone diagnostic mammography and any further action at this time; the implication is that the decision will be recon-

TABLE 5.3.
Expected Net Value for Strategies Using Hypothetical Net Benefits (in dollars)

Strategy	Net Value of Strategy[a]		Expected Net Value for $P(Ca)$	
	Women with Cancer	Women without Cancer	0.01	0.10
S_1	$-10,000$	0	-100^b	$-1,000$
S_2	$-50 - (0.7)(1,400) - 0.3(10,000)$	$-50 - (0.2)(900) - 0.8(0)$	-268	-340^b
S_3	$-50 - (0.7)(10,000) - 0.3(1,400)$	$-50 - (0.2)(0) - 0.8(900)$	-812	$-1,440$
S_4	$-50 - 1,400$	$-50 - 900$	-955	$-1,000$
S_5	$-50 - 10,000$	-50	-150	$-1,050$

[a] Numbers are rounded to the nearest whole number; expected net value $= P(Ca) \times$ net value for cancerous women $+ P(\overline{Ca}) \times$ net value for noncancerous women; $TP = 0.7$, $TN = 0.8$, $FN = 1 - TP$, $FP = 1 - TN$, $P(Ca) = 0.01$, and $P(\overline{Ca}) = 1 - P(Ca)$; net benefit of early detection $= -1,000$; net benefit of biopsy on false positive $= -500$; net benefit for missed cancer $= -1,000$; cost of mammography $= -50$; cost of biopsy $= -400$.

[b] Optimal, minimum-cost strategies for different risk groups.

sidered at some future time. Changing any of the numerical values assigned to the tree could alter the strategy choices in either of these circumstances. And one of the most important phases of analysis is thorough characterization of the sensitivity of choices to parametric variations. Although we stop short of that phase in this example, it was a major component of our work in the actual analysis of strategy alternatives presented in subsequent chapters.

Although the tree used in this example is artificially simple and the numbers are unrealistic, the basic ideas of decision analysis have been demonstrated. As a final note, all payoff values on the decision tree are negative because even in the best of circumstances there are substantial net costs associated with breast cancer. Positive benefits appear only briefly in time when breast cancer is detected early, providing a better prognosis as illustrated in one possible scenario in the next section; but on balance one faces aggregated net costs and reduced net costs, not net (positive) benefits.

BENEFIT-COST ANALYSIS

Benefit-cost analysis is usually perceived of as a methodology for evaluating and choosing among alternative public programs. Benefits and costs are projected for the lifetimes of competing programs. Nonmonetary benefits and costs are converted to dollar-equivalents by willingness-to-pay evaluations. Present, annual, or future equivalents are calculated for these benefit and cost flows using appropriate social discount rates (interest) to reflect societal views on the timing of benefits and costs.[2] Alternatives are compared on the basis of expected net benefits.

Standard measures of efficiency are used in program comparisons. The most appropriate measure is the net of discounted benefits less discounted costs. It is called the net present equivalent (NPE) when all costs and benefits have been converted to present equivalent values, the net annual equivalent (NAE) when costs and benefits have been annualized, and net future equivalent (NFE) when future equivalent values have been calculated for benefit-cost streams. A second measure, a very widely used one, is the ratio of discounted benefits to discounted costs. It is called the benefit-cost ratio B/C.[3] Present, annual, or future worths of benefits and costs may be used to calculate the ratio with identical results.

In contrast to the robustness of NPE, NAE, and NFE, great care must be exercised in defining benefits and costs if meaningful results are to be obtained using the B/C ratio. (The issue of measure selection is thoroughly discussed in Gohagan 1980.) For public programs benefits are the difference between the recipients' willingness to pay and what they actually pay. Economists refer to this difference as consumer surplus. Costs, on the other hand, consist of capital investment (adjusted for salvage when plant and capital equipment are involved), other first costs borne by society, and operating costs to the public provider of the benefit-generating service. If one mistakenly classifies cost savings as benefits or user fees as costs, the net equivalent measures are not affected, so program comparisons remain valid. But the B/C ratio can be seriously affected; in fact the ratio obtained is not the correct B/C ratio, and comparisons of alternatives are meaningless using such bastardized measures.[4]

Cost-effectiveness analysis is a variation on the same theme. When alternative actions can be presumed to offer equivalent benefits, one need consider only costs. Cost minimization is then the economic objective. When benefits can reasonably be measured only in nonmonetary terms like morbid days foregone, days of extended lifetime, or even numbers of morbid events, one can calculate the ratio of dollars expended per unit of benefit gained as an indication of cost effectiveness. But competing alternatives cannot be compared meaningfully on such mixed ratios unless the ultimate benefit of an additional day of life or one less day of morbidity is expected to be of the same magnitude for the alternatives. Examples of the potential problem of incomparable ratios are not hard to identify. There is always the possibility that a morbid day for a child may have incomparably different consequences than a morbid day for an adult. Also the loss of a child, in nonmonetary terms, is generally valued differently from the loss of an adult [Mishan 1978, OTA 1980].[5]

But benefit-cost and cost-effectiveness analysis need not be perceived as methodologies only for evaluating public programs. Both are valid procedures, with proper modifications in analytic perspective, for evaluating decision alternatives faced by either individuals or small groups. Naturally, costs and benefits must be identified and measured to properly reflect the perspective of the decision maker(s), and appropriate discounting practices must be employed. But the analytical process and the fundamental definitions of benefits and costs carry over.

We apply the concepts of benefit-cost analysis in our evaluations of alternative breast cancer detection strategies from the perspective of the individual. And we employ the more robust benefits-less-costs (NPE) measure of merit in lieu of the more popular ratio of benefits to costs. Our primary concern is the individual woman who must decide whether to undergo screening by whatever methods. Thus, most of our analysis is from her perspective. But insurance companies and the government cover the direct financial costs of most therapeutic and, in some instances, detection costs, so we also evaluate the alternatives from the perspective of the third-party payer.

Women have competing objectives to balance in making their choices regarding screening. They want to protect against early death and unpleasant morbidity from advanced breast cancer while avoiding unnecessary testing and surgery with their attendant direct and indirect costs. Third-party payers are (or perhaps we only wish they were) concerned with controlling costs subject to reasonable constraints on quality of care. The primary advantages seen by both parties are possibly extended disease-free lives. Women see possible psychosocial benefits plus economic advantages from early detection to be balanced against offsetting disadvantages of similar nature from unnecessary detection efforts and unnecessary biopsy in the event of false-positive findings. Third-party payers see offsetting advantages and disadvantages from early detection, false positive findings, and false negative examinations. Thus, each actor sees different possible net benefit flows from screening versus nonscreening alternatives.

The net benefit flows depicted in Fig. 5.2 are suggestive of what the two parties might perceive as the consequences of the C_8 and C_9 branches of the decision tree in Fig. 5.1. In contrast with the convenient round numbers previously assigned, these flows were chosen to reflect more plausibly the net of financial costs, psychological costs, and benefits of extended life as time progresses. An infinite variety of positive and negative flows are possible, depending on uncertainties in postdecision scenarios, but the timing and magnitudes shown are reasonable. These numbers presuppose that: procedural costs for treatment and therapy, and trauma, too, in the first two years are reduced by early detection; psychological costs fade with time as patients adjust to their changed lives and gain confidence in their health

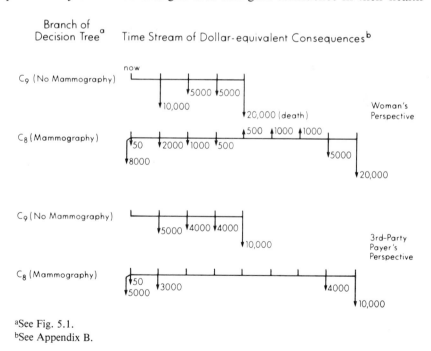

aSee Fig. 5.1.
bSee Appendix B.

Fig. 5.2. Comparison of hypothetical benefit-cost flows for an asymptomatic woman harboring a cancer, which will metastasize if not detected.

status, until recurrence or metastasis is detected; for long remissions there is a period of positive net benefits reflecting advantages of apparently disease-free living and reduced psychosocial and financial costs; and death is a close companion to recurrence or metastasis. The $50 charge at the beginning of the C_8 flow is for mammography. Women ordinarily bear this cost, but third-party payers might pay it if the marginal advantages outweighed the marginal costs, so it is included for both parties.

To evaluate the flows appropriate discounting rates should be applied as indicated previously. Choice of a discount rate for third parties, though not trivial, is relatively easy because all advantages and disadvantages are in dollar amounts, and third parties do have investment-rates-of-return requirements as standards. But it is more difficult to determine a suitable discount rate for individual women since many of their costs and benefits are psychosocial, and benefit-cost theorists are still at odds over whether discounting is even warranted. To circumvent problems of discount rate selection one typically evaluates the flows repeatedly using different rates, ranging, say, from 0 percent to 15 percent and investigates the selection implications of rate variation for more informed decision making. For each choice one calculates the net discounted costs (benefits are overpowered by costs in this example) and assigns the results to the decision tree. For each set of net discounted costs, the decision tree (Fig. 5.1) is reevaluated as in Table 5.3. Repeated reevaluations provide a basis for strategy selection.

STATISTICAL TECHNIQUES

Numerous statistical techniques were employed in the study. The main avenues of statistical analysis and the techniques utilized are depicted in Table 5.1. Discriminant analysis and logistic regression are illustrated in this section. Log-linear modeling of cross-classified categorical data is described briefly.

Discriminant analysis is similar to regression. One postulates a predictive equation (here called a discriminant function) incorporating variables presumed to have some discriminating value and calculates from the data the coefficients of the variables in the equation. It differs from regression in that the coefficients are calculated to maximize the discriminating power of the equation. Whereas in regression, values of the dependent variable are used with corresponding values of the independent variables to calculate the coefficients in the predictive equation, data for discriminant analysis are from two-way cross classifications.

Multivariate discriminant analysis provides better categorization of data than any single variable can when there is substantial overlapping of the distributions for individual variables within the categories [Hoel 1971]. A powerful form of discriminant analysis for model building is the stepwise version where the variables under consideration are entered and removed in stepwise fashion until a "best" function is obtained. A variable is included if its marginal statistical contribution to the discriminating power of the function is sufficient.

For two discriminating variables x_1, x_2 the discriminant function takes the form

$$y_j = a_1 x_{1j} + a_2 x_{2j}; \; J = 1, 2, \ldots, n$$

where subscripts 1 and 2 stand for groups, j is the identifier for individual datum within groups, and y is the projection of x values onto an inclined plane cutting through the x_1, x_2 plane (Fig. 5.3). The objective is to rotate the plane and find a_1 and a_2 so as to maximize the ratio of intergroup variation to intragroup variation. This provides maximum discrimination. The ratio to be maximized is

$$R = \frac{(\bar{y}_1 - \bar{y}_2)^2}{\displaystyle\sum_{j=1}^{n_1} (y_{1j} - \bar{y}_1)^2 + \sum_{i=1}^{n_2} (y_{2j} - \bar{y}_2)^2}$$

where $\bar{y}$ is the average value of x's projected on the inclined plane for each group, and y_{1j} is the projection of the jth member of the 1st group. Maximization is accomplished by equating to zero the partial derivatives of R with respect to a_1 and a_2 and solving the resulting linear equations for these constants

Consider the hypothetical data provided in Table 5.4. These data yield the following pair of equations to be solved for a_1 and a_2:

$$0.8 = 0.8 \, a_1 + 0.6 \, a_2$$

and

$$-0.4 = 0.6 \, a_1 + 1.2 \, a_2$$

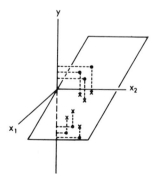

Fig. 5.3. Geometric depiction of projected data grouping in discriminant analysis.

TABLE 5.4.
Hypothetical Data for Two Discriminating Variables in Five Cases

		Observations (cases)				
Cancer cases	Spiculated mass, x_1	1	1	1	0	1
(Group 1)	Linear calcification, x_2	0	0	1	1	0
Noncancer cases	Spiculated mass, x_1	0	0	0	0	0
(Group 2)	Linear calcification, x_2	1	0	1	1	1

They are satisfied when $a_1 = 2.05$ and $a_2 = -1.34$. Hence, the discriminant function

$$y_j = 2.05 \, x_{1j} - 1.34 \, x_{2j}$$

This discriminant function can be used to classify other cases containing observations on the same variable. That in fact is the major value of the technique. Applied to the data in Table 5.5, the values y_j predicted for each group are as shown. Classification is achieved by choosing a threshold level for y_i and assigning every observation (case) with y_i above the threshold to the cancer group and every other case to the noncancer group. Different threshold levels produce different levels of accuracy in classification as shown in Table 5.5. For example, a threshold level of 0.01 correctly identifies 80 percent of the cancers and only 20 percent of the noncancers; this is a very sensitive but nonspecific classification rule. On the other hand, a threshold of 2.0 correctly identifies only 60 percent of the cancers but 80 percent of the noncancers; this is a less sensitive but much more specific classification rule. Final selection of the threshold level depends on the relative weights or aversions presumed for false negative and false positive examinations. This topic is further discussed in subsequent chapters wherever, in the context of analysis, it is appropriate.

To illustrate logistic regression, we will consider the data in Table 5.6. We use it to fit the following model (of log odds):

$$\ln \left[\frac{P(Ca)}{1 - P(Ca)} \right] = b_0 + b_1 \, x_1 + b_2 \, x_2$$

where x_1 is a "dummy" variable assuming the value $+1$ when a spiculated mass is present and -1 when no spiculated mass is present, and x_2 is a dummy variable coded $+1$ or -1 for presence or absence of linear calcification. The coefficients b_i are determined by the criterion of maximum likelihood; that is, they are chosen so that the probability of obtaining the observed data is maximized.

The maximum-likelihood computations are iterative and require several

TABLE 5.5.
Case Discrimination Using New Hypothetical Data

Observations (cases)

Cancer cases (Group 1)				
Spiculated mass, x_1	1	0	1	1
Linear calcification, x_2	0	1	0	1
Classification value, y_i	2.05	−1.34	2.05	0.71

Noncancer cases (Group 2)				
Spiculated mass, x_1	0	0	1	0
Linear calcification, x_2	0	1	1	1
Classification value, y_i	−1.34	−1.34	0.71	−1.34

	Correctly Classified as				Incorrectly Classified as			
	Cancer		Noncancer		Cancer		Noncancer	
Some threshold values for y_i	Number	Percent	Number	Percent	Number	Percent	Number	Percent
−1.3	4	80	3	60	2	40	1	20
0.01	4	80	1	20	4	80	1	20
0.7	4	80	1	20	4	80	1	20
2.0	3	60	4	80	1	20	2	40

TABLE 5.6.
Hypothetical Data for Logistic Regression

		Observations (cases)				
Cancer cases	Spiculated mass, x_1	1	1	1	0	1
	Linear calcification, x_2	0	0	1	1	0
Noncancer cases	Spiculated mass, x_1	1	0	0	0	0
	Linear calcification, x_2	1	0	1	1	1

steps to converge. We do not exhibit them here. The final result is the estimated (or fitted) logistic regression model

$$\ln\left[\frac{P(Ca)}{1 - P(Ca)}\right] = 0.134 + 1.234x_1 - 0.583x_2$$

The model predicts or estimates four conditional probabilities of cancer, depending on whether a spiculated mass or linear calcifications are present or absent. For example, if a spiculated mass is present and linear calcifications are absent, the estimated log odds is

$$\ln\left[\frac{P(Ca)}{1 - P(Ca)}\right] = 0.134 + 1.234(+1) - 0.583(-1) = 1.951$$

The odds of cancer can be obtained by exponentiating:

$$\text{Odds of cancer} = e^{1.95} = 7.036$$

And from this the probability can be calculated

$$P(Ca) = \text{probability of cancer} = 7.036/1 + 7.036 = 0.876$$

The four probabilities that can be estimated from the model are:

Spiculated Mass	*Linear Calcification*	*Probability of Cancer*
No	No	0.373
No	Yes	0.157
Yes	No	0.876
Yes	Yes	0.687

One can use the fitted logistic regression model as a diagnostic tool by choosing a cutpoint for the predicted probability and classifying all cases with higher probability in the positive category. Choice of the cutpoint affects sensitivity and specificity—the lower the value, the larger the sensitivity and the smaller the specificity.

Accuracy rates (sensitivity and specificity) for individual detection modalities and multimodality protocols can be calculated by applying logistic models to screening data. We do this in Chapter 7. Rates are more simply estimated from data that are cross classified by true disease state and test outcome.

Typically, data in cross classifications are not distributed proportionally. Log-linear modeling of such data yields a set of coefficients describing the departure from proportionality. Higher-order coefficients measuring variable interactions are small and typically not statistically different from zero. By setting these small coefficients equal to zero, one effectively borrows information from some cells of the classification table and shares it with other cells, thereby obtaining smoothed and more stable rate estimates.

The impact of log-linear smoothing is analogous to fitting a linear regression line to curvilinear data. The linear fit often yields more stable estimates of variable means than a more realistic curvilinear fit. In both cases the simplified model is a more convenient approximation to reality, making the best use of limited data.

We do not provide a simple example of log-linear smoothing here. The smoothing process itself introduces too much complexity for simple elaboration. We simply note that reference works are available [Mosteller 1968].

STRATEGY IDENTIFICATION AND EVALUATION METHODOLOGY

Whereas the techniques previously discussed are standard methods developed by others, the material presented in this section represents a new and original contribution to the fields of operations research and decision analysis. The techniques were developed by us for this research project. Only the essence of our method is discussed here. The details will be published in the appropriate technical literature.

A detection strategy can be thought of as a sequence of actions to be taken on the basis of test information at each step in the detection process. One must decide whether to do any testing at all and, subsequently, whether to do further testing, stop the process, or recommend a posttest course of action. The decision tree in Fig. 5.4 characterizes the situation for binary test outcomes.

The number of possible detection strategies grows astronomically as one increases the number of test modalities or the number of classifications of test results. For example, when test results are binary (positive or negative), there are 2 possibilities when no testing is done, 6 if only one test

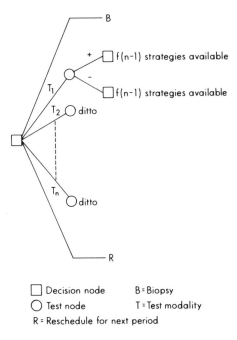

□ Decision node   B = Biopsy
○ Test node   T = Test modality
R = Reschedule for next period

Fig. 5.4. Abbreviated schematic of the decision tree for binary test outcomes.

possibility exists, 74 if two tests are available for use, and 16,430 if three tests are available. These numbers preclude retesting with a previously used modality; if retesting were permitted, that would further increase the number of strategy possibilties. But they include many strategies that incorporate actions contrary to test results as well as inefficient strategies that ignore the information obtained from some tests, as pointed out in the section on decision analysis.[6] Thus only a fraction of these possible strategies are viable contenders requiring analytical evaluation.

The recursive relations by which one determines the numbers of possible strategies are

n tests
Binary test results $f(n) = 2 + n\,[f(n-1)]^2$ $n = 0, 1, 2, \ldots$
Binary final actions

n tests
Binary test results $f(n) = k + n\,[f(n-1)]^2$ $n = 0, 1, 2, \ldots$
k-nary final actions $k = 1, 2, \ldots$

n tests
m-nary test results $f(n) = k + n\,[f(n-1)]^m$ $n = 0, 1, 2, \ldots$
k-nary final actions $k, m = 1, 2, \ldots$

Identification of viable contenders among these possible detection strategies requires a multifaceted systematic effort. All strategies not utilizing information generated by a test modality must be removed, for at least one other strategy not incorporating the unutilized test offers the same information at lower cost. Some such strategies are easily identified, but others are far more subtle, as shown in Fig. 5.5. In addition, strategies calling for intervention (for example, biopsy) on negative test results and doing nothing (for example, rescheduling a patient for reexamination in 12 months) on positive test results are senseless and must be removed.[7] When these considerations are accounted for, one finds that only a small fraction of possible strategies are viable contenders.

One needs to know more than how many viable strategies exist. One must know precisely which of the strategies are viable. With binary test results and final actions and up to three test modalities, 92 strategies are viable. Of these, 90, those incorporating tests, are shown in Fig. 5.6. Although we initially identified these strategies by inspection using the guiding principles discussed above, we have since developed a computer algorithm to produce the table, both for a check on the results obtained by hand and to provide a method that could be generalized as the need arose.

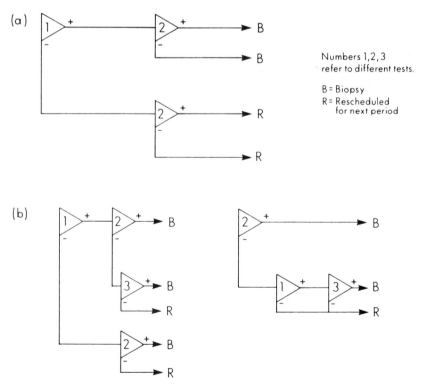

Fig. 5.5. Strategies not utilizing the information from a test.

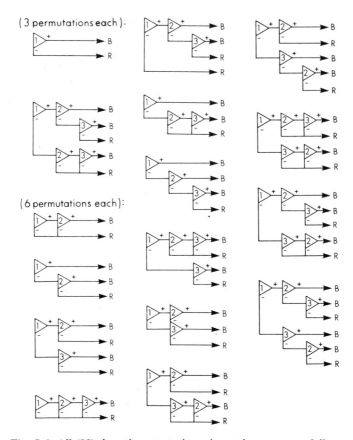

Fig. 5.6. All (90) detection strategies using at least one modality.

Once the viable strategies are enumerated, their evaluation proceeds via the methods of analysis illustrated in previous sections of this chapter. All of this is done by our strategy enumeration and evaluation algorithm.

Analytical results of our program can be plotted in the form of three-dimensional cost surfaces or tabulated to facilitate identification of optimal and suboptimal strategies for specific cost and diagnostic accuracy considerations. The selection process was illustrated for a hypothetical decision situation in the section on decision analysis. Three-dimensional plots are used in the strategy (protocol) analyses of Chapter 8.

NOTES

1. True positive and true negative rates for mammography are, respectively, the chance of a positive mammogram when cancer is present and the chance of a negative mammogram when there is no cancer. (Note that we use these terms as convenient synonyms for sensitivity

and specificity, whereas in many texts their meaning is different from this.) They must reflect actual clinical operations to be meaningful and can be estimated with reasonable accuracy from clinical data only if the clinic follows a fraction of both positive and negative cases for a long enough period to establish retrospectively their status at the time of examination.

2. Discounting is necessary to account for the time value of money. Even ignoring inflation, a dollar in hand is preferable to a dollar promised at some future date. Discounting is essential when program lifetimes are long. But over short periods of a couple of years or so, discounting is not as important since costs and benefits occur in close proximity and discounting will not likely alter their relative importance as it does when the two moieties are widely separated in time. The higher the discount rate, the more important is discounting.

3. Benefit-cost ratios are often misused in public sector analyses. The ratio here defined, the standard B/C, is useful only to the extent that alternatives for which B/C is less than zero are noncontenders from an economic perspective. The marginal ratio $\Delta B/\Delta C$, which measures the marginal advantage of more costly alternatives with possible greater benefits to less costly alternatives with different benefit levels, must be used to select among contending alternatives ($B/C \geq 1$). If the standard ratio B/C is used as the selection criterion, one might easily be led to select an alternative that violates the fundamental objective of maximizing net gain [Gohagan 1980].

4. These effects are not central to the work presented in this book. Although they are worth noting in passing, we leave it to the reader to seek numerical illustrations in methodological publications.

5. That humans hold divergent views regarding the relative worth of juvenile versus adult life under different living conditions is clear upon reflecting on the survivorship protocols of Eskimos and African bushmen in contrast with their attitudes in less stressful times. Whereas both peoples highly prize children, the very young are least valued and prime adults most valued when group extinction threatens. Although the perspectives of hunting and gathering societies are not those of more advanced societies like ours, the point of the observation is valid. The value of life depends on circumstances.

6. Enumeration of all possible strategies and identification of all viable strategies using up to three detection modalities was done initially by Gohagan and a research assistant, Valjean Spear. The recursive relation for counting strategies with binary test results and binary final decisions was specified by Spitznagel, who also wrote the computer programs for identifying, evaluating, and ranking all viable strategies.

7. These strategies would be sensible only if true positive rates for the tests utilized were smaller than false positive rates. But if this contrary situation existed, one would merely redefine positive and negative results so that true positive rates exceeded false positive rates.

REFERENCES

Fienberg SE (1977) The analysis of cross-classified categorical data. Cambridge, Mass, MIT Press.

Gohagan JK (1980) Quantitative methods for public policy. New York, McGraw-Hill, chaps. 18–21.

Hoel PG (1971) Introduction to mathematical statistics, 4th ed., New York, John Wiley and Sons.

Mishan EJ (1978) Cost-benefit analysis, expanded ed. New York, Praeger.

Mosteller F (1968) Association and estimation in contingency tables. J Amer Stat Assn 63:1–28.

U.S., Congress, Office of Technology Assessment (OTA) (1980) The implications of cost-effectiveness analysis of medical technology. Washington, D.C., OTA.

6

Risk Profiling

William P. Darby
John K. Gohagan
Edward L. Spitznagel

The predictive value of a detection modality is dependent on the accuracy of the modality (true positive and true negative rates) and the chance that the patient has the disease $P(C)$. The relationships are clear in the expressions for positive and negative predictive values, respectively:

$$P(C/+) = \left\{1 + (FP/TP)\,[P(\bar{C})/P(C)]\right\}^{-1}$$

and

$$P(\bar{C}/-) = \left\{1 + (FN/TN)\,[P(C)/P(\bar{C})]\right\}^{-1}$$

These are direct applications of Bayes' rule. Bayes' rule is the mathematical mechanism for revising probabilities on the basis of new (test) statistical information. Tests are calibrated in terms of true positive (TP) and false positive (FP) rates taking diseased and nondiseased patients as the bases.[1] Then a pretest estimate of the probability of disease, $P(C)$, is revised on the basis of test results using the first expression above, and the pretest probabilistic estimate for the absence of cancer, $P(\bar{C})$, is revised using the second expression [Gohagan 1980]. For example, if $FP = 0.61$, $TP = 0.68$, $P(C) = 0.003$, and $P(\bar{C}) = 0.997$, the chances that a positive test means cancer and a negative test means no cancer are 17 percent and 99.8 percent, respectively. But if $P(C) = 0.1$, the predictive values are 88 percent and 96.5 percent, respectively. These relationships are illustrated for a range of values in Table 6.1 (where it is clear that a combination of clinical examination and mammography provides the best predictive capability).

TABLE 6.1.

**Predictive Value by Disease Probability and Test Accuracy,
Illustrated with Data from BCDDP No. 25 (in percent)**

	Test Accuracy*		Predictive Value	
	True Positive	True Negative	Positive	Negative
Mammography	63	98	8.70	99.99
	38	99	10.30	99.98
Clinical palpation	26	99	7.30	99.88
	—	—	—	—
Thermography	21	95	1.25	99.87
	39	91	1.29	99.77
Clinical palpation and mammography	82	98	11.00	99.75
	68	99	17.00	99.90

Notes: P(C) = 0.003. Approximately 2 to 3 cancers per 1,000 women screened were detected at BCDDP No. 25. As *P(C)* increases, the predictive values increase for the same true positive and true negative values.

*These values are from Table 8.6. Pairs are given where it is not obvious as to which set of accuracy values is optimal.

The value $P(C)$ represents the chance that a woman has breast cancer at the time of the examination as estimated from pretest information. For asymptomatic women one has two choices for estimating $P(C)$: one can apply population-based disease rates, or one can differentiate on the basis of disease-related characteristics or features. The first alternative is nonselective and offers no advantage in terms of woman-specific predictability from test results. The second offers an opportunity to fine-tune the examination process to maximize the information gained from tests for individual women and minimize the chances of recommending biopsy needlessly or failing to recommend one that is needed.

Numerous epidemiological features have been implicated in the literature as risk modifiers (Table 6.2).[2] For example, many authors have argued that women who bear their first child while in their early twenties have a smaller lifetime chance of developing breast cancer than do women who postpone childbearing beyond the third decade of their lives. If lifetime risk is indeed modified by the presence of such features, one would also expect age-specific risk, $P(C)$, to be influenced, though not necessarily uniformly. And one would like to use this kind of information to calculate $P(C)$ for individual women or at least to classify women probabilistically as being low, medium, or high risk prior to testing. This would help determine which women should be examined regularly and would optimize test interpretation, as discussed above.

One of our objectives was to try to develop statistical risk profiles for women and to investigate the implications of risk level for test interpretation, examination protocol selection, and examination frequency. We reviewed

TABLE 6.2.
Risk Hypotheses from the Literature

Risk Feature	Presumed Direction of Correlated Lifetime Risk of Breast Cancer
Age	Positive
Female hormone intake (includes birth control pills)	Positive with extent of use
Female relatives with breast cancer	Strong positive correlation
Relatives with cancer	Positive correlation
Age at first pregnancy	Positive with age
Age at first birth	Positive with age
Number of pregnancies	Negative with number
Number of live births	Negative with number
Nursing history	Negative with duration
Age at menarche	Positive below age 12
Age at menopause	Positive above age 55
Prolonged menstrual history	Positive with duration
Fat consumption and obesity	Positive

the literature on risk and found most of it less than convincing and of little value in developing probabilistic risk profiles. (The major exception was the literature on radiation risk.) We also applied multivariate statistical techniques to Breast Cancer Detection Demonstration Project (BCDDP) No. 25 data and concluded that the really important risk modifier was age. BCDDP data cannot be used to assess radiation risk.

Our evaluations of risk data are summarized in the remainder of this chapter. The implications of risk variations for strategy selection are treated in Chapter 8 and those for examination frequency in Chapter 9.

CRITIQUE OF THE LITERATURE

We reviewed the literature in two phases.[3] In 1978 we concluded that published studies were of little value to practitioners in guiding decisions on the types and timing of examinations. There was practically no comparability among studies: population bases varied enormously, calculations of risk were done differently, and too little was specified regarding the sources and interpretations of the data to permit comparative analysis. The risk factors, derived by the authors as multipliers for scaling average risk to higher or lower risk, varied among studies by as much as an order of magnitude. Even for the same author one could not assess the importance of the simultaneous presence of more than one risk feature because the features were neither independent nor mutually exclusive and the degree of their statistical overlap was not assessed. Table 6.3 illustrates the variability found for some features.

In 1980 after analyzing BCDDP No. 25 data for risk implications we

TABLE 6.3.
Variability in Risk Factors from the Literature

Risk Feature	Variable Condition	Risk Factor*			
Previous disease	Benign	4.8	3.1	2.0	5.0
	Carcinoma	4.0	7.0	5.0	
Menstrual activity	Prolonged	1.4			
	Early onset	1.7			
Parity experience	Age at first birth $\geq$ 30	3.0	1.7		
	Total pregnancies $<$ 3	2.0			
	Never married	2.3	2.3	3.1	
Relatives with	Mother	2.0	3.0		
breast cancer	Sister	2.5			
	Mother and sister	15.0	47.0	5.10	

*For some features multiple risk factors have been reported in the literature as shown. A risk factor is a multiplier. For example, one writer argued that women with prolonged menstrual histories were 1.4 times more likely to develop breast cancer than women with menstrual histories of normal length.

again went to the literature. We chose 13 studies for critical review. We critiqued the latest and best studies we could find ignoring the issue of radiation risk at this point. Most of these studies contained enough data to check risk factor calculations and recalculate risk by other methods. Six of the studies covered numerous risk features, while the others were less extensive. Again we found substantial variability among studies. The general methodological approach was pairwise comparison of frequencies of presumed risk features in cancer and no-cancer populations. Statistical tests for significance were not widely employed, but a few authors did compute 95 percent confidence intervals to support judgments about the implications of their data [Brinton et al. 1979, Ross et al. 1980]. And two groups did use multivariate statistical techniques or direct controls on variables to help sort out the risk implications of individual features and groups of features [Brinton et al. 1979, Egan 1978]. Weaknesses observed were inadequate sample sizes, nonrandomness in sampling, lack of control over intervening variables when investigating the impacts of another, and omission of data pertaining to the feature under discussion. Most of the 13 studies suffered from one or more major shortcomings in data or technique. But even so, the data bases and methods of analysis were clearly superior, in most instances, to those we found in 1978.

We computed risk factors from data provided in these studies by the three methods shown below as illustrated in Table 6.4.

R_b = risk level in relation to some baseline risk level, B

$$= \frac{P(\text{feature level } L/C) \div P(\text{feature level } L/\overline{C})}{P(\text{feature level } B/C) \div P(\text{feature level } B/\overline{C})}$$

R_r = relative frequency of a feature in cancer, C, and noncancer $\overline{C}$, cases

$$= \frac{P(\text{feature } /C)}{P(\text{feature } /\overline{C})}$$

R_m = cancer frequency among patients with a feature compared to the overall population

$$= \frac{P(C/\text{feature})}{P(C)}$$

The baseline risk ratio R_b was commonly used in the papers reviewed as was the relative risk ratio R_r. The risk factor needed for modification of normal or average epidemiological risk is R_m. We found substantial variation of each ratio depending on the data source. But the variability was less than recorded in the 1978 review. Differences ranged from 20 to 30 percent for

TABLE 6.4.
Example of Alternative Risk Factor Calculations Using Age
at First Childbirth as the Feature

Age at first birth	Total	Breast Cancer		Risk Factor*		
		Yes	No	R_b	R_r	R_m
Less than 20	620	150	470	0.44	0.57	0.67
20 to 24	1,208	388	820	0.65	0.84	0.89
25 to 29	827	332	495	0.93	1.19	1.12
30 or more	514	225	289	1.08	1.38	1.32
Nulliparous	762	320	442	1.00	1.29	1.17
Total	3,931	1,415	2,516			

*The base level for calculating relative risk R_b is nulliparous women. For example, for the age range 20 to 24 years:

$$R_b = \frac{388/820}{320/442} = 0.65$$

Source: Data from Paffenbarger et al. 1980.

women bearing children late to 200 to 300 percent for women whose mothers had breast cancer. Comparisons for age at first childbirth are shown in Fig. 6.1. Also see Table 6.4.

Once again, we did not find in the published literature convincing numerical estimates of relative risk by risk feature. Some authors thought

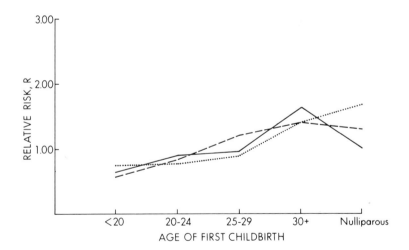

.... Sartwell et al. 1977
‒ ‒ ‒ Paffenbarger et al. 1980
─── Brinton et al. 1979

Fig. 6.1. Baseline relative risk, R_b, for age at first childbirth.

they saw strong links between disease frequency and certain features, while others did not. The root of these differences appeared to lie in the populations selected for study. But we concluded from our critique of these publications that substantially increased risk associated with a family history of breast cancer was certainly plausible and that although late first childbirth and early menarche or late menopause may increase risk slightly, the increase would not be enough to influence decisions regarding examination frequency or protocol selection. The major impact of age as a risk feature was apparent in all studies and in all age-specific incidence rates reported.

RADIATION RISK

Another potentially important risk feature is frequency of previous breast X rays. Ionizing radiation of all kinds definitely causes chromosomal damage. Some of the damage is repaired in the cell nucleus before replication. But some damage results in mutations that are carried on by cell mitosis and may produce cancerous growths. It has been shown in laboratory studies that cancer rates among experimental animals can be increased even with low levels (a few rads) of X-radiation [Hall 1978]. And epidemiological studies have documented higher breast cancer rates among women exposed to 50 rads or more of radiation from atomic explosions, fluoroscopy, and radiation therapy [Boice et al. 1979, Upton et al. 1977]. Since fractionation studies have shown that repeated low doses are ultimately as carcinogenic as a single exposure of the aggregated dosage, and modeling of empirical data from the epidemiological studies supports linearity of risk with dose, one can only conclude that even diagnostic mammography carries some radiation risk, especially when frequently repeated [NCRP 1980]. (The critical issue is not risk but the benefit-risk balance — see Chapter 9.)

ANALYSIS OF BCDDP NO. 25 RISK DATA

The National Cancer Institute (NCI) collected especially detailed risk feature data for 150 of the BCCDP No. 25 participants. These women were interviewed extensively in a controlled study for the purposes of risk evaluation. This group, representing part of the population included in the work of Brinton et al. [1979], consisted of three age-matched subgroups: 51 women who developed cancer in the five years of the project, 57 disease-free women who had had a breast biopsy for suspicious findings while participating in the project, and 42 participants who never had a biopsy and were disease free up to the time of the interview. These would have been excellent cases for study, but numbers and resulting statistical power were so small for this group that no statistical significance could be found for any risk feature. Hence, these detailed histories are not incorporated into our analysis.

BCDDP No. 25 collected data on most of the risk features listed in Table 6.1 for the 10,187 women screened in the form of medical histories provided by each participant upon entry into the program and updated at each subsequent screening visit. (See Appendix A for history data collection forms.) The following discussion is based on analyses of those data.

We began with pairwise comparisons of feature frequencies among women diagnosed with breast cancer and those who remained disease free. Sample sizes and achieved significance levels are given in Table 6.5. Some of the features that appear to have statistical significance are age confounded and completely disappear after age correction. For example, younger women are not as likely to have aunts with breast cancer as are older women. Older women are less likely to have used birth control pills because the pill was not available during their reproductive years. Younger women tend not to have undergone menopause yet. Age at menarche is difficult to remember accurately, and periodic recollections among participants vary by a year or so. The popularity of breast feeding is age confounded. Consequently, these pairwise results are at best suggestive. They are certainly not conclusive.

Multivariate discriminant analyses of these data controlling for age were run. When the effect of age was removed, none of the other epidemiological features was a significant contributor to risk.[4] Thus, the only risk feature of real significance in BCDDP No. 25 data is age.

One might argue that the entire BCDDP No. 25 population is at high risk and feature discrimination would be unlikely. Without controls we cannot pass final judgment. However, tumor rates seem comparable with those reported for the nation, and the population does exhibit good variability on most risk features. Therefore, we think we would have found strong risk-influencing features in our data analysis if they existed. Weaker risk features will typically be found only when the number of cancers is very high, such as in case-control studies, and should not affect screening decisions.

CONCLUSION

We conclude from our critique of the literature and our analysis of BCDDP No. 25 data that the premier risk feature is a woman's age. It is the only feature of significance in BCDDP No. 25 data. A family history of breast cancer, especially if more than one female member of a family had the disease, would seem to be a probable second important risk feature. Such a pattern could be environmentally or genetically linked. But we are not convinced by the literature that the statistical link is especially strong, and BCDDP No. 25 data are inadequate to test the relationship.

Another feature of apparent significance appears to be previous ex-

TABLE 6.5.
Pairwise Statistics for BCDDP No. 25 Risk Data

Variable by Category	Achieved Significance	No Cancer	Cancer	Total
Female relative(s) had breast cancer	—	1,491(27.6)	156(26.9)	1,647(27.5)[a]
Grandmother(s) had breast cancer	—	795(3.5)	132(4.6)	927(3.7)[a]
Mother had breast cancer	—	802(5.5)	132(6.8)	934(5.7)[a]
Sister(s) had breast cancer	—	601(3.7)	129(3.9)	730(3.7)[a]
Aunt(s) had breast cancer	—	815(11.9)	132(6.3)	947(11.4)[a]
Daughter(s) had breast cancer	—	321(4.7)	8(0.0)	329(4.6)[a]
Family history of cancer	—	543(83.8)	50(90.0)	593(84.5)[a]
Ever taken birth control pills	0.0007[b]	1,007(23.6)	153(9.8)	1,160(21.8)[a]
Ever taken famale hormones	—	580(59.0)	16(43.8)	596(58.6)[a]
Age at menarche	0.0937[c]	582(13.1)	70(12.7)	652(13.1)[d]
Age at menopause	0.0135[e]	1,265(45.6)	136(47.3)	1,401(56.8)[d]
Number of years between menarche and menopause	—	356(33.2)	60(34.2)	416(33.4)[d]
Age at first pregnancy	—	514(23.1)	54(23.5)	568(23.5)[d]
Age at first birth	—	510(24.5)	53(24.5)	563(24.5)[d]
Number of live births	—	549(2.6)	77(1.6)	626(2.5)[d]
Number of unsuccessful pregnancies	—	549(0.5)	77(0.5)	626(0.5)[d]
Total months of breast feeding	0.007[c]	513(6.9)	80(3.5)	593(6.4)[d]

[a]Percentage of population with this factor.
[b]Absence of factor associated with cancer.
[c]Low values associated with cancer.
[d]Average value of variable in the subpopulation.
[e]High values associated with cancer.

posure of the breasts to ionizing radiation. There are no data from BCDDP No. 25 on this variable. But the literature is scientifically convincing. Although the level of risk for doses as low as 1 rad is unknown, available data on large-dose effects are consistent with a linear model, and low-dose risk has been estimated by extrapolation by a number of groups to be on the order of 3.5 to 6.5 additional cancers $\times$ 10^{-6} rad^{-1} yr^{-1} for life after a latency period of 10 years.

Because age so clearly dominates as a risk modifier — and is the only one we could confirm in BCDDP No. 25 data — we do not employ multiattribute risk profiles in subsequent chapters to directly estimate $P(C)$. Instead we use age-specific incidence data to make a first estimate of $P(C)$ and parametrically modify it to test for the sensitivity of results for possible risk-influencing features as appropriate in the analysis of alternative detection protocols and examination schedules. (See Chapters 8 and 9.) We incorporate the potential for radiation risk into our models separately because the risk-benefit balance of mammography is a key consideration in protocol selection and examination scheduling.

NOTES

1. The false positive rate for the test, *FP*, is the estimated probability that the test will be positive when cancer is not present, $P(+/\overline{C})$. The true positive rate, *TP*, is the estimated probability that the test will be positive when cancer is present, $P(+/C)$. The true negative rate or estimated specificity of the test is just $(1 - FP)$. The false negative rate is related to the true positive rate, or estimated sensitivity, by the expression $FN = 1 - TP$.

2. By epidemiological risk features we mean aspects of a woman's personal history that are not related to previous breast disease. Previous breast disease, especially previous breast cancer, places a woman in a substantially higher risk category.

3. Much of this section is based on work done by Rita Menitoff and John Goodman under the supervision of John Gohagan.

4. We also incorporated a number of features to represent history of breast disease. These were previous breast infection, lumps, pain, skin changes, and bloody nipple discharge. Only skin changes remained significant when age was controlled for, and this is more a symptom, than a feature. Thus, these variables do not appear in our risk analysis for asymptomatic women.

REFERENCES

Boice JD, Land CE, Shore RE, Norman JE, Tokunaga M (1979) Risk of breast cancer following low-dose radiation exposure. Diagnostic Radiology 131:589–597.

Brinton LA, Williams RR, Hoover RN, et al. (1979) Breast cancer risk factors among screening program participants. J Natl Cancer Inst 62:27–43.

Carlile T. (1981) Breast cancer detection. Cancer 47:1164–1169.

Cole, P, Elwood JM, Kaplan SD (1978) Incidence rates and risk factors of benign breast neoplasms. Am J Epidemiology 108: 112–120.

Craig TJ, Comstock GW, Geiser PB (1974) Epidemiologic comparison of breast cancer patients with early and late onset of malignancy and general population controls. J Natl Cancer Inst 53:1577–1581.

Davies DF, Torng A, Morris EB, Sebes J (1978) Estimates of composite risk factors for death from breast cancer. J Natl Ca..cer Inst 61:41–48.

Egan RL (1979) Estimated risk and occurrences of breast cancer in asymptomatic and minimally symptomatic patients. Cancer 43:871–877.

Egan RL, Mosteller RC, Stephens CD, Egan KL, (1977) Risk, biopsy, and breast cancer: new approach through combined epidemiologic, clinical, and X-ray indications. Breast, Diseases of the Breast 4:, n.p.

Gohagan JK (1980) Quantitative methods for public policy. New York, McGraw-Hill, chap. 18.

Hall EJ (1978) Radiobiology for the radiobiologist, 2nd ed. Hagerstown, Mo., Harper & Row.

Lilienfeld AM, Coombs, J. Bross IDJ, Chamberlain A (1975) Marital and reproductive experience in a community-wide epidemiological study of breast cancer. Johns Hopkins Medical J. 136:157–162.

MacMahon B, Cole P, Brown J (1973) Etiology of human breast cancer: a review. J Natl Cancer Inst 50:21–42.

Menitoff R (1978) A decision analytic approach to the evaluation of alternative breast cancer practices and strategies. Masters thesis. Sever Institute of Technology, School of Engineering and Applied Science, Washington University, St. Louis, Mo.

Miller AB (1981) Breast cancer. Cancer 47:1109–1113.

National Council on Radiation Protection and Measurements (NCRP) (1980) Mammography Recommendations of the National Council on Radiation Protection and Measurements. NCRP no. 66. Washington, D.C., NCRP.

Ory, H. Cole P, MacMahon B, Hoover R (1976) Oral contraceptives and reduced risk of benign breast diseases. New Engl J Med 294:419–422.

Paffenbarger RS, Jr., Kampert JB, Chang H (1980) Characteristics that predict risk of breast cancer before and after the menopause. Am J Epidemiology 112:258–268.

Ross RK, Paganini-Hill A, Gerkins VR, et al. (1980) A case-control study of menopausal estrogen therapy and breast cancer. JAMA 243:1635–1639.

Sartwell PE, Arthes FG, Tonascia JA (1977) Exogenous hormones, reproductive history, and breast cancer. J Natl Cancer Inst 59:1589–1592.

Shapiro S, Strax P, Venet L, Fink R (1968) The search for risk factors in breast cancer. Am J Public Health 58:820–834.

Upton AC, Beebe GW, Brown JM, et al. (1977) Report of NCI Ad Hoc Working Group on the risks associated with mammography in screening for the detection of breast cancer. J Natl Cancer Inst 59:481–493.

Vessey MP, Doll R, Sulton PM (1972) Oral contraceptives and breast neoplasia: a retrospective study. Br Med J 3:719–724.

Vorherr H (1980) Breast cancer: epidemiology, endocrinology, biochemistry and pathology. Baltimore-Munich, Urban and Schwarzenberg.

7

Predictive Capabilities of Test Modalities

John K. Gohagan
Edward L. Spitznagel
William P. Darby

Two types of information were recorded for each test modality. Abnormal breast features observed during palpation or on mammographic or thermographic images were recorded individually.[1] The clinicians and radiologist interpreters additionally recorded their diagnostic interpretations of the examination information and made recommendations for appropriate medical action. For example, the mammographer might conclude that a mass or cluster of punctate calcifications observed on the X-ray film probably represented a malignancy and should be biopsied for definitive diagnosis. Data reflecting examiners' diagnostic interpretations and recommendations we call diagnostic and recommendations data to distinguish these data from the more basic, less subjective features data. We use the two groups of data separately in evaluations of the technical capabilities of the three modalities employed in screening.

We calculate true positive and true negative rates for individual interpreters of Breast Cancer Detection Demonstration Project (BCDDP) No. 25 directly from the diagnostic and recommendations data.[2] The more basic features data we use to develop statistical models for predicting disease and formulating biopsy recommendations without regard for the actual final diagnostic interpretations and recommendations of the examiners. With this two-leveled approach to evaluation we can contrast the performance of human interpreters as individuals with statistical models to gain insight into what, if any, accuracy advantages might be associated with either of the two different approaches.

The analysis is presented in three stages. We begin by listing a variety of reasonable definitions for positive and negative examinations. These we developed from the diagnostic and recommendations options available to the examiners on the standard data collecton forms. For each set of definitions sensitivity and specificity rates are calculated for individual modalities and multimodality protocols by cross-tabulating disease status at the time of examination against test results. These rates provide an indication of the technical capabilities of each test modality as it was used at BCDDP No. 25. More important, they provide a quick, easy-to-comprehend look at how test accuracy varies with alternative definitions of a positive test.

In the second stage, using the same diagnostic and recommendations data, we develop statistical models for predicting disease. The tools employed are multivariate discriminant and regression analyses. In this way we develop optimal definitions of positive and negative examinations for each modality and for combinations of modalities. The rates found by this method include those obtained from the cross-tabulations but suggest no significant opportunities for improved definitions.

In the third stage we develop additional statistical models for test interpretation. Here we use only the more basic features data. Increased accuracy rates for individual modalities are not obtained in this stage of analysis even though the features considered to be the primary predictors of disease by the examiners are the features in the model. This suggests that examiners may be using information not incorporated in the features as they were recorded on the standard data collection forms. It does turn out, however, that the statistical model has normative value as a guide to which cases should be biopsied.

DISEASE FEATURES, DIAGNOSES, AND RECOMMENDATIONS

The features variables observed upon examination, as well as possible examiner interpretations of those features, are summarized in Tables 7.1, 7.2, and 7.3. The features data include size, shape, location, and other information pertaining to mass(es) palpated during physical examination or observed on the film images; distribution, size, and shape of microcalcifications observed on mammograms; and location and source of temperature asymmetries observed on thermograms. Diagnoses and recommendations options available to examiners range from suspected malignancies and recommended biopsy to negative examinations with neither biopsy nor aspiration recommended.

EMPIRICAL ACCURACY: CROSS-TABULATED DIAGNOSTIC DATA

Accuracy rates vary with the definition of a positive examination. The instant one tries to tabulate statistics on the ability of an examination

TABLE 7.1.
Physical Features and Diagnostic Variables for Clinical Exam

Feature

Mass(es) present	Breast characteristic
Right or left	Nodularity
Location(s) in breast	Small, large
Diameter dominant mass	Thickening
Texture dominant mass	Diffuse, localized
Hard, soft, cystic	Retraction
Mobility dominant mass	Skin changes
Movable, fixed deep or skin	Axillary nodes, palpable
Shape dominant mass	Nipple changes
Discrete, irregular	

Interpretation

Diagnosis right and left	Recommendation
Mass(es) right and left	Months to next exam
Review of case at conference	
Breast distortion: benign, malignant	Biopsy:right, left, both
Degree of confidence	Aspirate:right, left, both

modality to detect disease (sensitivity) and sort out negative cases (specificity), one faces the problem of defining positive and negative test results. The more restrictive the definition of a positive examination, the less sensitive and more specific the modality appears. Less restrictive definitions make the modality appear more sensitive.

Because of this trade-off relationship between sensitivity and specificity, it is essential to calculate both rates for each definitional option for comparison. Many definitions are possible using the standard diagnostic and recommendations options available to examiners on BCDDP standard forms. For instance, one might define a positive mammogram as one for which a malignancy was suspected and biopsy was recommended. Or one might define it so loosely as to include observation of a shadow of undetermined nature for which the woman was placed on an accelerated reexamination schedule. Seven credible definitions of positive examinations are given in Table 7.4. A typical example of appropriately cross-classified data is given in Table 7.5. These frequencies were generated by applying definitions *A* to the screening data. True positive and true negative rates for all seven definitions are given in Table 7.6.[3]

Among the alternative definitions, none is clearly dominant in the sense that all others produce both inferior sensitivity and specificity rates. The definitions of positive examination *D* are clearly best for clinical palpation. None of the others offer superior sensitivity without excessive sacrifices in specificity.[4] The choice of definitions is not so clear-cut for thermography, mammography, or the two-modality protocol incorporating

TABLE 7.2.
Image Features and Diagnostic Variable for Mammography

Feature	
Mass(es) present	Nonvascular calcification
Right or left	Shape
Number	Punctate, ring, linear, large con-
Location dominant mass	glomerate
Location second and third masses	Distribution
Marginal characteristics dominant	Multiple, scattered, linear,
mass	clustered
Spiculated, ill versus well defined	Architectural distention
Marginal characteristics second and	Location in breast
third masses	Distribution
Shape dominant mass	Localized, diffused
Oval or round, multinodular,	Breast characteristic
spiculated or stellate	Size, diameter
Shapes second and third masses	Skin thickening
Diameter dominant mass	Localized, diffuse, areolar
(two views)	Retraction
Diameter second and third masses	Nipple changes
	Retraction, enlarged, inverted

Interpretations	
Diagnosis right and left	Recommendation
Normal	Months to next exam
Mass(es):benign, malignant	Review of case at conference
Calcification:benign, malignant	Biopsy:right, left, both
Dysplasia	Specified mass(es) calcification(s)
Architectural distortion:benign,	Architectural distortions, or
malignant	Increased densities
Increased density:malignant	Aspirate:specified mass(es)
Degree of confidence	

both clinical palpation and mammography. Definitions *D* and *E* are equivalent for mammography, yielding $TP = 63$ percent and $TN = 98$ percent. But definition *A* offers superior specificity (99 percent) with some sacrifice in sensitivity (58 percent), and it is not immediately obvious which is preferable. Finally, definitions *A* and *C* are equivalent for the two-modality protocol, $TP = 68$ percent and $TN = 99$ percent, but *D* offers much improved sensitivity (82 percent) with one point less specificity (98 percent).

When trade-offs between sensitivity and specificity are required, choices depend on implicit—or, preferably, explicit—assignments of weighting factors to both false negative and false positive examinations, because the choice requires preferentially sacrificing sensitivity for compensating (nonlinear) gains in specificity or vice versa. Thus, it would appear that the best definitions among those specified in Table 7.4 are *D* for clinical palpation, *A* for thermography, and either *D* or *F* for mammography, depending on one's preference for false positive or false negative errors.

TABLE 7.3.
Image Features and Diagnostic Variables for Thermography

Feature

Asymmetric background temperature	Asymmetric vascular pattern
Right, left, both	Right, left, both
Location	Location
Distribution	Cause
Diffuse, localized	Increased vein:caliber, number, temperature

Interpretation

Diagnosis right and left	Recommendation
Normal versus abnormal	Months to next exam
Degree of confidence	Review of case at conference

TABLE 7.4.
Alternative Definitions of Positive Test Results with Accuracy Rates— Diagnostic and Recommendations Variables Only

A
$C+$ = biopsy
$M+$ = biopsy
$R+$ = biopsy
$T+$ = review[b]

B
$C+$ = malignant
$M+$ = malignant
$R+$ = biopsy
$T+$ = abnormal[c] and review

C
$C+$ = malignant or biopsy
$M+$ = malignant or biopsy
$R+$ = biopsy
$T+$ = abnormal and review

D
$C+$ = biopsy or[a] recall
$M+$ = biopsy or recall
$R+$ = biopsy or recall
$T+$ = (abnormal and[a] review) or recall

E
$C+$ = biopsy or aspirate or recall
$M+$ = biopsy or aspirate or recall
$R+$ = biopsy or aspirate or recall
$T+$ = (abnormal and review) or recall

F
$C+$ = malignant or biopsy or aspirate or recall or review
$M+$ = malignant or biopsy or aspirate or recall or review
$R+$ = biopsy or aspirate or recall
$T+$ = (abnormal and review) or recall

G
$C+$ = malignant or biopsy or aspirate or recall or review
$M+$ = malignant or biopsy or aspirate or recall or review
$R+$ = biopsy or aspirate or recall
$T+$ = abnormal or review or recall

[a]*And* means both; *or* means one or both.
[b]*Review* means review the entire medical record at a conference of all examiners.
[c]"Abnormal" was the only diagnostic category.

TABLE 7.5.
Cross-Tabulation of Positive and Negative Test Results by Actual Disease State

Case Status	Test Outcomes Using Outcome Definitions A								Total
	T–M–C–	T–M–C+	T–M+C–	T–M+C+	T+M–C–	T+M–C+	T+M+C–	T+M+C+	
Not biopsied[a]	67,756	71	80	4	6,714	13	17	5	74,660
Negative biopsies[b]	174	50	103	8	51	25	24	3	438
Cancer diagnosed[b]	22	8	27	5	11	2	20	7	102[c]
Total	67,952	129	210	17	6,776	40	61	15	75,200

[a]Breasts not biopsied are labeled positive on the basis of the elements of the definitions even though in the actual screening the final decision was not to biopsy. See Table 7.4 for definitions.

[b]Biopsies recommended by BCDDP No. 25 and those done on the basis of examinations conducted on participating women at other locations between screenings are included. Follow-up data were available for all cases.

[c]The true positive rate for mammography under the definitions is approximately 57 percent (100 × 59/102).

Note: Tabulation is by breast, not by woman.

TABLE 7.6.

True Positive and True Negative Rates for Alternative Definitions of Positive Examinations (in percent)

| | Definitions | | | | | | | | | | | | |
| | A | | B | | C | | D | | E | | F | | G | |
	TP	TN	TP	TN	TP	TN	TP	TN	TP	TN	TP	TN	TP	TN
Mammography	58	99	50	99	58	99	63	98	63	98	71	95	71	95
Clinical palpation	22	99	15	99	23	99	26	99	25	99	41	64	41	64
Thermography	39	91	20	95	21	95	43	73	43	73	43	73	57	25
Clinical palpation and mammography*	68	99	59	99	69	99	82	98	74	97	86	61	86	61

*This strategy of doing both tests and recommending biopsy if either is positive is the best of the two-modality strategies under a wide range of conditions. See Chapter 8.

Notes: Strategy selection requires assigning relative weights to TP and TN rates to reflect perspectives on the adverse nature of missed cancers and unnecessary biopsies. For example, if a missed cancer is considered to be 10 times worse than an unnecessary biopsy, the weighted sum of the two rates for mammography and clinical palpation under definitions D would be: wtd. sum(M) = $1/11(10 \times 63 + 1 \times 98) = 66$; wtd. sum (C) = $1/11(10 \times 26 + 1 \times 99) = 33$. Equivalent numbers for definitions F would be 73 and 43, respectively. In this instance the TP rates are the key considerations making both modalities appear to be better under definitions F than D, with mammography the better of the two modalities. As the weighting ratio increases from 10:1 to, say, 1000:1, the preference for mammography increases and definitions F becomes increasingly appropriate. The opposite is true as the weighting ratio decreases to, say, 1:10, with clinical palpation becoming preferable under definitions D. See Table 7.4 for definitions of positive and negative examinations.

One could as well tackle the problem of selecting among alternative definitions of a positive test by assigning weights at the outset and comparing definitions on the basis of average weighted accuracy. Table 7.7 illustrates the trade-off relationships for the definitions in terms of alternative weighting schemes. Average weighted accuracy was calculated from the relation.[5]

$$\text{Wtd Accuracy} = (w_1 \times TP) + (w_2 \times TN)$$

When $w_1:w_2$ is larger than 10:1, F is the best set of definitions for positive test results. When the weights are set at 1:1, the desirability rankings for rules vary; for example, definitions D are best for clinical palpation and mammography, while A is best for thermography. As w_2 is increased further to reflect the desire to avoid false positive results, the definitions with the highest true negative rates are increasingly preferred.

One could conclude from an extension of this third analysis that one particular set of definitions was better than the others in specified circumstances, but it would not be valid to presume that selection to be universally best, especially since other definitions are possible. However, the implications of alternative selections for test accuracy are clearly portrayed in the previous discussion. In subsequent sections these implications are not so obvious in the analysis—that is why we presented them here in some detail.

One might expect the accuracy rates for the individual modalities to be age dependent because breast characteristics change dramatically with age. Age-specific true positive and true negative rates are given in Table 7.8 and do appear to show age-specific variations. However, this is an artifact of statistical variation due to small sample sizes. In fact, in the age ranges of BCDDP No. 25 women, accuracy rates are essentially constant, as indicated by the rates calculated following log-linear smoothing, also shown in Table 7.8.

REESTIMATION OF ACCURACY
VIA LOGISTIC REGRESSION

The analysis presented in the previous section is insightful in that the implications of alternative definitions of positive and negative tests in terms of false negative and false positive examinations are made clear. However, multivariate statistical regression and discriminant analysis techniques are more incisive and thorough means of establishing definitions of positive tests when sufficient data are available. Our objective in this second stage of analysis is to distinguish statistically between cancerous and noncancerous cases. This is a simple binary distinction, with a low frequency of cancer cases. Therefore, one must use a technique specifically designed for a categorical response variable. After some experimentation logistic regression

TABLE 7.7.
Weighted Averages of True Positive and True Negative Rates

	Definitions[a]													
	A		B		C		D		E		F		G	
$W_1:W_2$[b]	10:1	1:1	10:1	1:1	10:1	1:1	10:1	1:1	10:1	1:1	10:1	1:1	10:1	1:1
Mammography	61	76	55	74	61	78	66	81	66	81	73	83	73	83
Clinical Palpation	29	61	23	57	30	61	33	63	32	62	43	53	43	53
Thermography	43	65	27	58	28	54	46	58	46	58	46	58	54	41
Clinical Palpation and mammography	71	84	63	79	72	84	83	90	76	86	84	74	84	74

[a] Definitions are provided in Table 7.4.
[b] W_1 = weight for true positive rate. Large W_1 reflects distaste for cancers missed. W_2 = weight for true negative rate. Large W_2 reflects desire to avoid negative biopsies.

TABLE 7.8.

**Age-Specific True Positive and True Negative Rates before and after
Log-Linear Smoothing of Data, Definitions *A* (in percent)**

	Age Range					
	36-46		47-56		57 and up	
	TP	TN	TP	TN	TP	TN
Before smoothing						
Mammography	46	99	44	99	66	99
Clinical palpation	30	99	15	99	23	99
Thermography	46	89	26	91	44	92
After smoothing						
Mammography	59	99	58	99	58	99
Clinical palpation	23	99	22	99	21	99
Thermography	46	89	40	91	38	92

Note: Definitions *A* for positive examinations are given in Table 7.4.

was found to be appropriate, and a linear function of the following form
was therefore fitted to the diagnositc and recommendations data:

$$\ln\left[\frac{P(C)}{P(\bar{C})}\right] = b_0 + b_1 x_1 + \ldots + b_n x_n$$

The probabilities $P(C)$ and $P(\bar{C})$ are for cancer and no-cancer, respectively.
And, although not shown explicitly, they are conditional on the features
observed on examination. The x's are the individual diagnostic and recommendations variables or features described previously and are assigned
values of 1 or 0 depending on whether they were observed by the examiner
on a particular examination.

The analysis was done in steps because of the large number of variables
and cases involved. First, univariate analyses were done to identify the
variables that, alone and interactively with others, were statistically predictive. Nonpredictive variables and interactions were eliminated from further
consideration, although certain variables thought by clinicians to be important were forced into the analysis and maintained unless they were found
unequivocably to be statistically noncontributors.[6] This reduced set of
variables constituted the starting set for the logistic regression.

Regression models for individual and combined modalities were then
developed using half of the data (half of the medical records in our data
base). These cases were selected randomly to represent the whole population
of medical records. The models specified were then applied to the unused
half of the data to test their ability to classify cases correctly as cancer and
no-cancer and thereby calculate sensitivity and specificity rates.

Finally, coefficients for these models (the same variables) were recalculated using the whole population of cases. These coefficients are more representative of BCDDP No. 25 data and more stable than those calculated from the split sample. The variables incorporated in the final models are those obtained in the split-sample analysis just described because no additional variables were found to be statistically significant when the full complement of cases was considered.

For any set of variables observed on examination, the logistic regression equation has a particular numerical value, k. The corresponding probability of cancer for the individual examined is

$$P(C) = \frac{e^k}{(1 + e^k)}$$

Thus defining a positive examination in terms of certain diagnostic and recommendations variables (the x's) is tantamount to defining it in the terms of the calculated probability $P(C)$ that cancer is present [Cox 1970].

Sensitivity and specificity rates are directly related to $P(C)$. Setting the threshold level too high results in frequent failure to biopsy existing cancers. Setting it too low means frequent biopsies of noncancerous breasts. Sensitivity and specificity rates for individual modalities are plotted in Fig. 7.1.

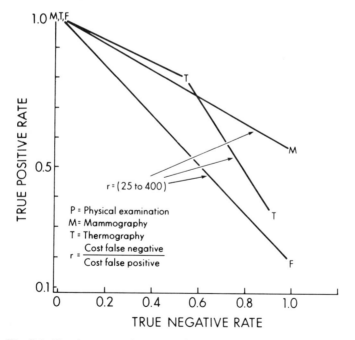

Fig. 7.1. Receiver operating curves for modalities using diagnostic and recommendations data.

Those for combined modalities are plotted in Fig. 7.2.[7] Selected points on the curves are marked with a cost ratio, the cost of a missed cancer per unit cost of false positive biopsy. These costs that increase monotonically from right to left along the curves provide a guide for selecting operating points.

Working backward through the analysis, we conclude the following. First, sensitivity and specificity rates for mammography are higher than for either clinical palpation or thermography. Clinical examination is more sensitive but less specific than thermography. Second, thermography in combination with either or both of the other modalities contributes nothing of statistical significance to accuracy and could be of value only in instances where findings on the other two modalities were at odds—although even then its value seems doubtful—or when the objective is to avoid mammography for fear of radiation hazard.

The best combination of modalities on the basis of this analysis using diagnostic and recommendations data is therefore clinical palpation and mammography, which confirms previous observations in the cross-tabulation analysis. We cannot push this phase of analysis further. To identify the best malignancy-predicting features, we must use the features data.

PREDICTIVE ACCURACY USING OBSERVED PHYSICAL EXAM OR DIAGNOSTIC IMAGE FEATURES

Concentration on the actual features observed during examination, in lieu of the integrated judgments of examiners as in the previous two sections, introduces greater objectivity and generalizability into the analysis. Here again, the multivariate statistical techniques of discriminant analysis and logistic regression are employed. The same three-phased variable selection and model development process previously discussed is followed, including split-sample analyses to estimate sensitivity and specificity rates. Plots of sensitivity versus specificity are given in Fig. 7.3 and 7.4.

The best model for discriminating between malignant and benign cases incorporates clinical palpation and mammography. This is consistent with previous findings. In the optimal logistic regression model, 15 variables from the two modalities are incorporated. These are listed in Table 7.9 with their coefficients. Only one interaction term appears in the list, although all interactions were tested for; the other interactions are not good statistical predictors.

With this model one accumulates the screening information for asymptomatic women. If in any examination during a one- or two-year period any one of the variables listed in Table 7.9 is detected, that variable is to be counted as present for biopsy decisions at each subsequent examination in that period. Whenever a combination of variables has been observed so that the appropriate sum of the model coefficients is -3.5472 or larger, biopsy is in order.[8]

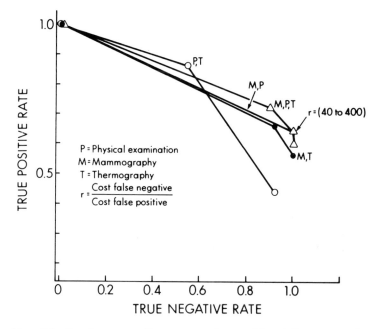

Fig. 7.2. Receiver operating curves for multimodality protocols using diagnostic and recommendations data.

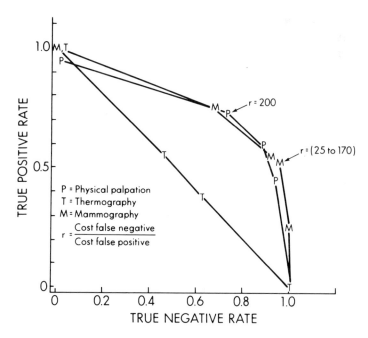

Fig. 7.3. Receiver operating curves for modalities using features data.

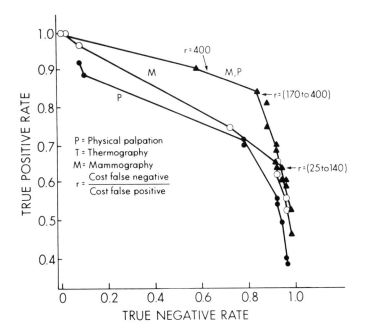

Fig. 7.4. Receiver operating curves for multimodality protocols using features data.

The log odds of malignancy for a set of observed features are calculated as follows. Record each feature (Table 7.9) observed on palpation and mammography. Add the coefficients for each feature observed. Subtract the coefficients for all features not observed. (For the interaction term, add the coefficient 1.217 if the features are simultaneously present or absent. Subtract it if only one is present.) The result is k = log odds. For example, if none of the specified features are observed on palpation but clustered punctate calcifications are observed on mammography, the sum, including the constant, is -1.914 for the physical exam variables. For mammography the sum is

$$-2.112 - 0.346 + 1.341 + 0.354 + 1.217 - 1.221 = -0.767$$

for a total of $k = -2.681$. Since this is greater than -3.5472, biopsy is in order.

If this rule is observed consistently in a clinical setting, true positive and true negative rates of 53 percent and 98 percent will be achieved for asymptomatic women. This is the best one can do using only features variables and a linear model. This is not as good as definitions A (Table 7.6) in which a positive test means that a biopsy is recommended. But the rates in Table 7.6 are accurate only to within about 10 percent, so that the discrepancy is not so great as it might appear initially. On the other hand,

TABLE 7.9.
Logistic Regression Coefficients for Disease Features Model

Variable X_i *	Coefficient, b_i†
Physical Exam	
Mass	2.935
Immobile mass	2.128
Hard-textured mass	−1.619
Cystic-textured mass	−2.290
Irregular-shaped mass	1.451
Small marbly nodularity	−0.323
Minor nipple changes	−0.416
Skin retraction or nipple retraction	0.355
Mammography	
Irregular, spiculated, stellate mass	2.112
Ill-defined edges of mass	0.346
Punctate calcifications	1.341
Clustered calcifications	0.354
Interaction between clustered and punctate calcifications	1.217
Localized architectural distortion	1.221
Constant	0.307

*All interactions were considered. These are the only significant features.

†Negative signs indicate greater likelihood of benign disease, and positive signs indicate greater likelihood of malignancy. To determine log odds of malignancy for any given set of features, add all coefficients together with signs reversed for those features not present. (For the interaction term add the coefficient 1.217 if the features are simultaneously present or absent. Subtract it if only one feature is present.) Using −3.5472 as a cutoff valve, corresponding to biopsy if the likelihood of malignancy is at least 2.8 percent, yields sensitivity of 53 percent and specificity of 98 percent.

the discrepancy does exist, and this suggests that the examiners were able to use information not incorporated in the features variables.

SUMMARY OF FINDINGS

Results of the three approaches to estimating the predictive capabilities of modalities require different interpretations.

Analysis of diagnostic and recommendations data by cross-tabulation yields true positive and true negative rates depicting actual performance at BCDDP No. 25 under various definitions of a positive examination. These results are accurate to within about 10 percent. A final choice on operating definitions for clinical palpation and mammography for positive examinations cannot be made from this analysis without assigning relative weights or preference values to true positive and true negative (or false positive and false negative) examinations because selection requires trading off sensitivity for specificity.

Reanalysis of the same data using logistic regression confirms the accuracy of the tests as calculated by cross-tabulation but offers no normative insight into how better to define positive examinations.

Analysis of the more objective features data provides a normative basis for deciding when to recommend biopsy but does not yield higher accuracy rates than the best possible rates observed in the cross-tabulations. The inability of statistical optimization to match the raw tabulated rates suggests that information other than what is contained in the features data was utilized by examiners. We do not know what that information was; it is worth repeating that the regression model included all variables thought to be important by the examiners. The result of this analysis can be applied in other clinical settings as illustrated in the text using Table 7.9.

NOTES

1. Recall that physical examinations were done by one of two nurse practitioners with oversight provided by a senior surgeon. (See Chapter 3.) All thermograms were read by a radiologist specializing in thermography. All mammograms were read by a different radiologist specializing in mammography. No information about the woman under examination was available to an examiner other than the findings with his or her examination modality. The radiologists worked only from films—they did not even see the woman.

2. Sensitivity and specificity rates estimated from diagnostic and recommendations variables are unavoidably interpreter specific. Since interpreters integrate in their minds the image data or physical features observed in the process of formulating a diagnosis and recommendation, one cannot extricate their judgment from the observed data. Because in our study one interpreter read all mammograms while another read all thermograms, the rates we calculate from these data measure the performance of these interpreters working with the technology and technicians available at BCDDP No. 25. Rates for clinical examination reflect the average performance of two nurse practitioners. The nurse practitioners and radiologist thermographer performed at about the levels generally achieved in other clinical centers, judging by published data. The radiologist mammographer performed well above the average, judging from rates published by other BCDDPs [Hicks 1979, Mahoney 1979].

3. Sensitivity (*TP*) reported in an earlier publication was for definitions *F*. At that time we did not have an adequate sample of cases with all negative examinations, so that we could not accurately calculate specificity rates (*TN*). The rates in Table 7.6 are stable.

4. One must keep the true negative rate very high to avoid excessive biopsy rates. A true negative rate of 99 percent means that on each visit 1 percent of the noncancer subpopulation will be sent on for biopsy. In five visits of the same subpopulation approximately 5 percent of its members would be biopsied. On an individual basis this is tantamount to an *n* percent chance of a noncancerous woman being biopsied in *n* years of annual examinations.

5. Nonlinear relationships are possible. For example, one could define a utility function over the two variables (x = sensitivity and y = specificity) and plot a surface $u(x,y)$. Under certain very restrictive conditions the utility function is linear: $u(x,y) = u(x) + u(y)$. Under somewhat more realistic conditions it may be quasi-linear: $u(x,y) = u(x) + u(y) - k\, u(x)\, u(y)$. For individuals it might even be possible to assess $u(x)$ and $u(y)$. However, from a practical perspective linear weighting is usually preferable.

6. Chi-square levels in this analysis are inflated by our using a random sample of cases for women never biopsied and having to scale these data to represent the entire population of never-biopsied women. This is required because we use 100 percent samples for biopsied and cancer cases. When these data are scaled to represent all cases never biopsied, it swells the apparent sample size substantially, and chi-square values increase with sample size *n* since

$$\chi^2 = \sum_{\substack{i \\ \text{groups}}} \frac{n(P_i - p_i)^2}{P_i} \; ; \quad \begin{array}{l} p_i = \text{observed proportion} \\[4pt] P_i = \text{expected proportion} \end{array}$$

7. Plots of this type are often referred to as receiver operating curves (ROC) in deference to their origin in communications theory. The usual ROC plot shows sensitivity against one-minus-specificity or TP versus FP.

8. Optimal sensitivity ($TP = 53$ percent) and specificity ($TN = 98$ percent) with this model (that is, the features data) are achieved if biopsy is recommended when $P(C)$ reaches 2.8 percent. This corresponds to a log odds of

$$k = \ln(0.028/0.972) = -3.5472.$$

REFERENCES

Cox DR (1970) The analysis of binary data. London, Methuen.

Dixon WJ, Brown MB (eds) (1979) Biomedical computer programs (BMDP). Health Sciences Computing Facility Department Biomathematics, School of Medicine, UCLA. Los Angeles, University of California Press.

Hicks MJ, Davis JR, Layton JM, Present AJ (1979) Sensitivity of mammography and physical examination of the breast for detecting breast cancer. JAMA 242:2080–2083.

Mahoney LJ, Bird BL, Cooke GM (1979) Annual clinical examination, the best available screening test for breast cancer. New Engl J Med 301:315–318.

Nie NH, Hull CH, Jenkins JG, Steinbrenner K, Bent BH (1975) Statistical package for the social sciences (SPSS), 2nd ed., New York, McGraw-Hill.

8

Strategy Selection

Edward L. Spitznagel
John K. Gohagan

A detection strategy is a set of instructions specifying the actions to take at each step of the detection process from initial test selection to the final decision on biopsy. Each choice depends on the age-specific epidemiology of disease, previous test results, the technical capabilities of tests, and cost implications under specific disease conditons. For example, a hypothetical strategy incorporating three tests (or examination modalities) is to begin the detection process with clinical palpation, do a mammogram if palpation is negative (otherwise biopsy the palpated lesion), biopsy if the mammogram is positive, do a thermogram if the mammogram is negative, biopsy on a positive thermogram, and reschedule the woman for her next periodic examination if the thermogram is negative. The first step in strategy selection is identification of all possible viable strategies incorporating up to three test modalities (clinical palpation, mammography, and thermography) [Gohagan 1980].

IDENTIFICATION OF VIABLE STRATEGIES

In Chapter 6 a recursive function was given for counting the maximum possible number of strategies for up to three test alternatives with binary results (negative/positive) and binary final-action alternatives (biopsy/reschedule for periodic examination). The recursive function for n tests was given as

$$f(n) = 2 + [f(n - 1)]^2$$

so that with $f(0) = 2$, $f(1) = 6$, $f(2) = 74$, and $f(3) = 16,430$ possible strategies.

The detection process for which this recursive function is applicable actually begins prior to any testing. Prior (to tests) information including age, possible symptoms, and epidemiological risk features is used to decide whether to apply a first test modality. Before any testing is done three options exist. These are to forego all testing and biopsy on the basis of prior information, to terminate the examination process and reschedule the woman for a future examination, or to apply one of the three detection modalities to obtain additional evidence to help confirm or disconfirm the presence of cancer. Basically, the same options are available upon observing the results of the first and second tests. But following the third test, the only options are biopsy and reschedule for a future examination.[1]

Only 92 of the 16,430 strategies require detailed analysis. All others either are equivalent to 1 of the 92 or are dominated by 1 or more of them. As an example of equivalence the two strategy groups shown in Fig. 8.1 can be shown to be equivalent by rediagramming the first. In this instance equivalence depends on the fact that the diagnostic tests were done independently, so that the order in which tests are done is not important. In situations where independence is not maintained, which is typical of most diagnostic practices, order would be important, of course, and these two strategies would not be equivalent.[2]

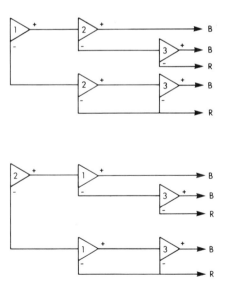

Fig. 8.1. Two equivalent strategies. Numbers in triangles specify test modalities. Each diagram represents a group of six strategies, since test numbering may be permuted. The symbols *B* and *R* stand for biopsy and reschedule for a future examination, respectively.

Within the set of all unique strategy possibilities there is a partial ordering, which we call dominance. When two strategies *A* and *B* use the same level of diagnostic information but strategy *B* is more costly, strategy *A* is said to dominate. Thus strategies not utilizing the information generated by one of the incorporated modalities are dominated by otherwise equivalent strategies that do not include that modality. Two examples of this situation are provided in Fig. 8.2. The second example is subtle, but reformatting shows that modality 1 is ignored when modality 2 is positive. Strategies like that in Fig. 8.3 calling for biopsy upon negative test results and rescheduling for a future reexamination upon positive tests results are "illogical" and dominated by strategies that are identical except that they call for the opposite actions on the basis of the same information. Dominance is implied by the fact that true positive rates (*TP*) calculated from our data exceed false positive rates, raising the cost of the first strategy group.

The set of all viable strategies is given in Fig. 8.4.

EVALUATION AND SELECTION METHODOLOGY

Expected cost per screen is the desirability indicator used in this analysis. Financial costs associated with individual tests, biopsy, and therapeutic

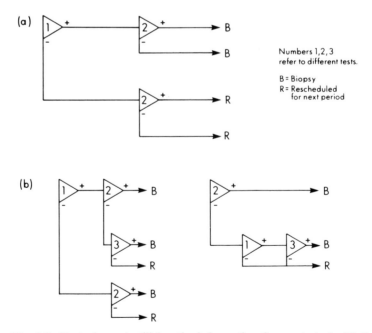

Fig. 8.2. Strategies not utilizing the information from a test. In **(b)** the left strategy is dominated by the strategy to the right.

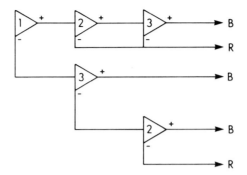

Numbers 1,2,3 represent different tests.
B = Biopsy
R = Reschedule for next period

Fig. 8.3. An illogical strategy when *TP* > *FP*.

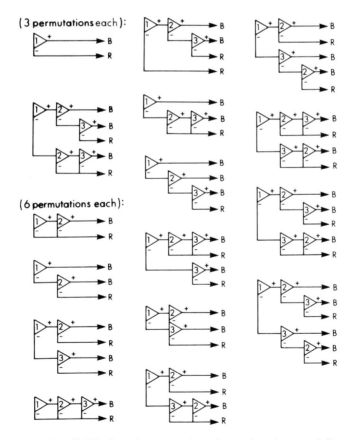

Fig. 8.4. All (90) detection strategies using at least one modality.

surgery are accounted for. These are derived from financial data from the Washington University Medical Center as representative of ordinary practice settings and from Breast Cancer Detection Demonstration Project (BCDDP) No. 25 screening cost data as representative of high-volume, very efficient screening centers. Psychosocial costs for false negative and false positive examinations, on the other hand, are situation specific and cannot be accurately estimated. These are incorporated into the analysis parametrically to permit wide-ranging evaluations of the sensitivity of strategy rankings to their magnitudes. (Cost estimation is the topic of Appendix B.)

Two additional factors included in the evaluations are radiation hazard from X-ray mammography and increased risk of breast cancer with age. Radiation risk has been estimated by epidemiologists and medical physicists as individual scientists and as members of National Cancer Institute and UN working groups. The estimates range between 3.5 and 7.5 additional cancers per million women exposed per rad of radiation [Boice et al. 1979, UNSCEAR 1976, Upton et al. 1977]. These estimates are still imperfect, especially regarding very low-dose exposures, and do not easily translate into dollar-equivalent costs per mammogram, so they are incorporated parametrically.[3] We accounted for the age dependency of breast cancer rates directly from BCDDP No. 25 screening data by reworking the analysis for women in three age groups: 36 to 46, 47 to 56, and 56 years or above.[4]

Benefits are incorporated as negative costs or cost savings. Thus the best strategy in a given set of circumstances is the one with the lowest expected cost—with costs adjusted to reflect the particular circumstances.

The probabilities required for the calculations are the eight probabilities p_i ($i = 1, \ldots, 8$) of obtaining each of the possible test outcome combinations (ranging from all three tests negative to all three positive) and the conditional probabilities Cp_i ($i = 1, \ldots, 8$) of malignancy for each possible combination of test outcomes. We obtained these probabilities by fitting what is referred to as a "parsimonious" log-linear model involving five variables—age group, presence of malignancy, and the outcome of each of the three tests—to the corresponding frequencies from BCDDP No. 25 screening data. Probabilities so obtained are more reliable than rates calculated directly from observed frequences because a nonsaturated log-linear model makes use of information from other cells in cross-tabulations of disease state by test findings to adjust out the instability of low-frequency cells. We used the log-linear models program BMDP3F to identify strong and weak interactive effects. Then we suppressed the weak interactive effects (forced to zero) and estimated the p_i and Cp_i values needed. This method has already been used with substantial success in the National Halothane Study [Bunker et al. 1969, Mosteller 1968].

The calculational burden associated with evaluating and rank ordering 92 strategies would be substantial without an efficient algorithm. Although each of the 92 nondominated strategies can be represented as a decision tree, computerization in the form of numerical arrays is more efficient. Thus the strategies are represented as four, eight-element arrays of 0's and 1's with 0 representing reschedule for future examination and 1 indicating performance of a test or biopsy. Three of the arrays are for the three different tests, and the fourth is for biopsy decisions.

The eight elements in each array correspond to the eight possible outcomes of the tests *as if* all three tests are done, even though in most strategies fewer than three are actually performed, and never are all three performed all of the time. By (our) convention the eight positions in the arrays are ordered from all tests negative to all tests positive.

As an example of the array representation of a strategy, consider one where subsequent tests are done only if the preceding test(s) were negative, and biopsy is recommended if any test is positive.[5] Such a strategy and its corresponding array are given in Fig. 8.5.

Expected cost calculations, exclusive of the costs associated with missed cancers and unnecessary biopsies for this strategy, are easy to make in matrix form; one merely takes the product of a matrix and two vectors:

$$E^*(\text{cost}) = \begin{pmatrix} \text{cost} \\ \text{vector} \end{pmatrix} \times \begin{pmatrix} \text{test results} \\ \text{and biopsy} \\ \text{decision matrix} \end{pmatrix} \times \begin{pmatrix} \text{product} \\ \text{probability} \\ \text{vector} \end{pmatrix}^t$$

$$= [C, M, T, B] \times \begin{bmatrix} 1 & 1 & 1 & 1 & 1 & 1 & 1 & 1 \\ 1 & 1 & 1 & 1 & 0 & 0 & 0 & 0 \\ 1 & 1 & 0 & 0 & 0 & 0 & 0 & 0 \\ 0 & 1 & 1 & 1 & 1 & 1 & 1 & 1 \end{bmatrix} \times \begin{bmatrix} P_{---} \\ P_{--+} \\ P_{-+-} \\ P_{-++} \\ P_{+--} \\ P_{+-+} \\ P_{++-} \\ P_{+++} \end{bmatrix}$$

The asterisk is included to signify the absence of psychosocial costs in the calculations.

The expected costs of false positive biopsy decisions and false negative decisions (failure to biopsy a carcinogenic breast) are calculated separately and added to the expected costs calculated as above to obtain the total expected cost of a strategy. For example, the expected cost of a false positive examination with the strategy in Fig. 8.5 is

$$E_{FP}(\text{cost}) = \begin{pmatrix} \text{cost of} \\ \text{false} \\ \text{positive} \end{pmatrix} \times \begin{pmatrix} \text{biopsy} \\ \text{decision} \\ \text{vector} \end{pmatrix} \times \begin{pmatrix} \text{product} \\ \text{probability} \\ \text{vector} \end{pmatrix}^t$$

$$= (FP, \text{dollars}) \times [0\ 1\ 1\ 1\ 1\ 1\ 1\ 1] \times \begin{bmatrix} P_{---} \times CP_{---} \\ P_{--+} \times CP_{--+} \\ \vdots \\ P_{+++} \times CP_{+++} \end{bmatrix}$$

Similarly, the expected cost of a false negative examination is

$$E_{FN}(\text{cost}) = (FN, \text{dollars}) \times [1\ 0\ 0\ 0\ 0\ 0\ 0\ 0] \times \begin{bmatrix} P_{---} \times (1 - CP_{---}) \\ P_{--+} \times (1 - CP_{--+}) \\ \vdots \\ P_{+++} \times (1 - CP_{+++}) \end{bmatrix}$$

Note that calculations for the two kinds of error require complementary decision vectors and conditional probabilities.

Because three of the most important costs involved, those of false negative and false positive biopsy decisions and of radiation hazard, are known only within very broad limits, they are treated as parameters to be varied, as indicated earlier. Strategy comparisons are accomplished by repeated evaluations over the ranges of parameters, and results are presented parametrically. In this way broad ranges of parameter values are identified in which particular strategies are optimal. Only a few of the 92 strategies were found to be optimal within the entire range of parametric values employed.

RESULTS

Some of our results are displayed in the perspective drawings of Figs. 8.6 and 8.9. Overall expected cost for minimum-cost strategies is plotted

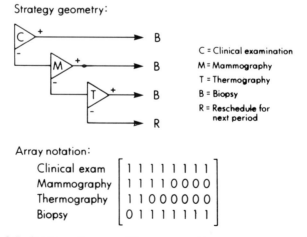

Fig. 8.5. Strategy diagram with corresponding array representation.

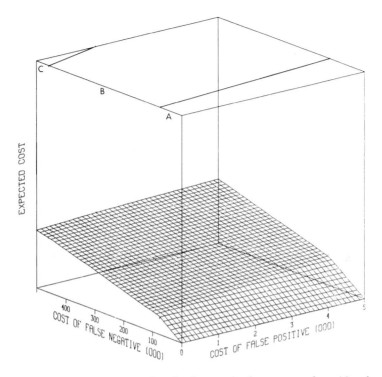

Fig. 8.6. Expected costs and optimal strategies for women of age 46 and under where biopsy cost is $600 and each examination costs $60.

against wide-ranging values of total possible financial and psychosocial costs for incorrect biopsy decisions. Each planar surface on the maps corresponds to a different strategy. The folds in the cost surfaces are the boundaries at which two strategies have equal expected cost; these boundaries have been projected onto the top sides of the reference cubes and the corresponding regions labeled to indicate the optimal strategies.

Age is a major consideration in selecting a strategy. Figs. 8.6 through 8.8 illustrate this by giving optimal costs and strategies for three age groups; 46 and below, 47 to 56, and 57 and above. Cost per screening modality was set at $60 per woman, and cost per biopsy was set at $600. Both false positive and false negative scales in the figures are in units of $1,000. (Computations were done per breast or side, using $30 per examination, rather than per woman in order to utilize screening data properly.)

In each of the figures three strategies occur as optimal under certain circumstances. Those strategies are:

A — perform no tests and no biopsies;
B — perform a mammogram and biopsy if it is positive; and
C — perform a mammogram first, and biopsy if it is positive;

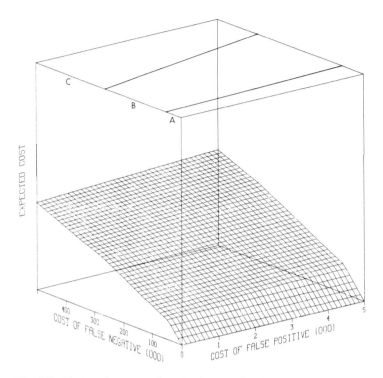

Fig. 8.7. Expected costs and optimal strategies for women of ages 47 to 56 when biopsy cost is $600 and each examination costs $60.

if it is negative, perform a physical examination and biopsy if it in turn is positive.

These strategies, along with the others occurring in Figs. 8.9 through 8.11, are diagrammed in Fig. 8.12. In the foreground of Figs. 8.6 to 8.8 strategy *A* is optimal. This region corresponds to low-risk aversion, with cost of testing and biopsy being the largest component of expected cost. In that region expected cost can be minimized by performing no tests at all. As expected, that region is largest for the low-prevalence group of Fig. 8.6 and smallest for the high-prevalence group of Fig. 8.8.

The next strategy in Fig. 8.6 through 8.8 moving out along the surfaces is *B*, mammography alone followed by biopsy if it is positive. In this region the cost of a false negative is sufficiently high that testing is justified; and as might be expected, the test indicated, mammography, was the one that our data showed as having the greatest precision. The third strategy consists of a combination of mammography and physical examination, with biopsy when either is positive. The truly optimal strategy *C* is to do mammography first, with the physical examination performed if the mammogram is

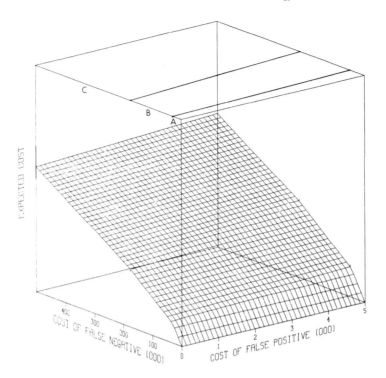

Fig. 8.8. Expected costs and optimal strategies for women of age 57 and above where biopsy cost is $600 and each examination costs $60.

negative. Another strategy with the two tests reversed has practically the same expected cost, and a third strategy in which both tests are always performed is only slightly more costly. The latter strategy is probably the kind of simplified strategy that would be adopted for sound practical reasons.

With increasing age of women, and correspondingly increasing prevalence, strategies *B* and *C* tend to move closer to the foreground, indicating that higher-risk women in general should be examined by mammography or mammography in combination with clinical palpation.

Radiation risk, too, is a critical factor in strategy selection. Although 3.5 to 7.5 cancers per year per million women per rad of radiation seems a small number, this is a cumulative phenomenon, and the cancers generated are in women who in the absence of radiation would not have developed the disease.

Radiation risk has the effect of raising the cost of mammography, with the amount of increase related to dosage level and the rate of tumor generation per rad. Because these factors are imprecisely known, one must perform strategy selection over a broad range of increased mammography cost possibilities. For the medium-prevalence group, ages 47 to 56, originally

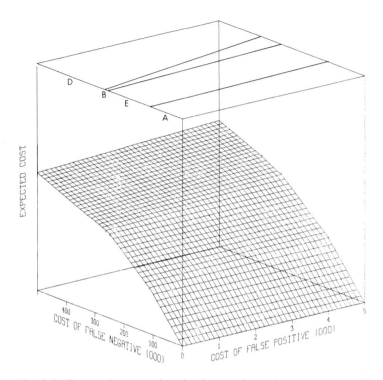

Fig. 8.9. Expected costs and optimal strategies under the same conditions as in Fig. 8.7 except mammography costs have been raised to $240 to include radiation risk.

shown in Fig. 8.7, the following happens as mammography costs are increased. First, with very little increase in cost the background region of strategy *C* switches to strategy *D*, namely,

> *D* — perform a physical examination first and biopsy if it is positive; if it is negative, perform a mammogram and biopsy if it in turn is positive.

This is a minor change, coming about primarily because strategy *D* avoids mammography in a small fraction of cases.

When mammography cost reaches approximately $120, including longterm radiation risk and examination charges, a new, more complex strategy, *E*, is inserted in a narrow band between strategies *A* and *B*:

> *E* — perform thermography first; if positive, do a physical examination; if physical is positive, biopsy; if physical is negative, do mammography; if mammography is positive, biopsy.

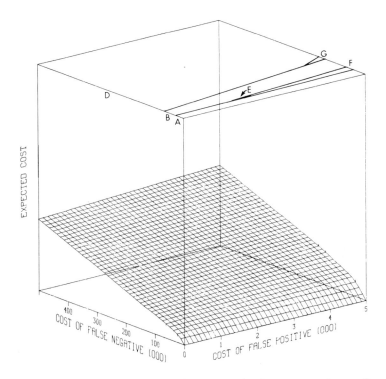

Fig 8.10. Expected costs and optimal strategies for women of ages 47 to 56 when biopsy cost is $600 and costs of physical examination, mammography, and thermography are $10, $20, and $10, respectively.

The effect here is to use thermography as an initial screen to reduce the number of mammograms substantially. As the cost of mammography is increased even more, the strategy *E* region widens substantially. For a multiattribute (including radiation risk) cost of $240 per mammogram, the cost surface is given in Fig. 8.9. In addition to the wide region for strategy *E*, there is also a widened region for strategy *A*, in which no tests are performed, indicating that higher potential costs dissuade women from screening.

Large-scale, efficient screening centers such as the BCDDPs can make all three test modalities available at substantially lower costs than those assigned above. For women aged 47 to 56, Fig. 8.10 shows cost surfaces and optimal strategy regions for a mass screening system in which physical examination and thermography are each $10 per woman, and mammography is $20 per woman. This is in total a cost of $40 per woman for all three tests, which is roughly what the BCDDP No. 25 costs have run.

Again, the familiar strategies *A*, *B*, and *D* appear, with the region for *D* coming much farther forward and regions for *A* and *B* being much more

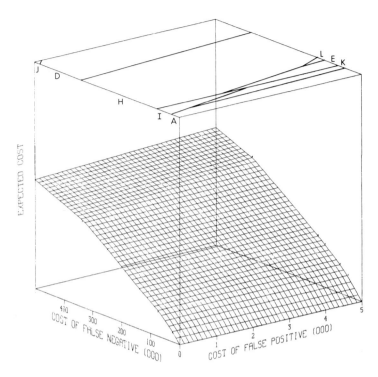

Fig. 8.11. Expected costs and optimal strategies under the same conditions as in Fig. 8.10 except mammography costs have been raised to $240 to include radiation risk.

narrow. Thus, when tests are less expensive, even the moderately risk averse find them advantageous.

In addition to the strategies, *A*, *B*, and *D*, two strategies *E* and *F* that use thermography as a prescreen to cut down on use of mammography appear between regions *A* and *B*. The basic reason for their appearance is that mammography is more expensive than thermography. Also a small wedge of strategy *G*, which is like strategy *C* except that it requires thermographic confirmation of physical examination, occurs in a wedge between regions *B* and *D*. That region corresponds to individuals who are highly averse to false positive examinations and moderately averse to false negative examinations. For diagrams of all strategies occurring in these figures, see Fig. 8.12.

In Fig. 8.10 we have seen the effect of low-cost screening with mammography slightly more expensive than the other tests. If the cost of mammography is increased to reflect radiation risk, much the same thing happens as described earlier except that strategy *B* disappears completely at approximately an $80 cost of mammography and is replaced primarily by strategy *H*, which is like strategy *D* except that here again thermography is used as a prescreen for mammography, though not for physical examina-

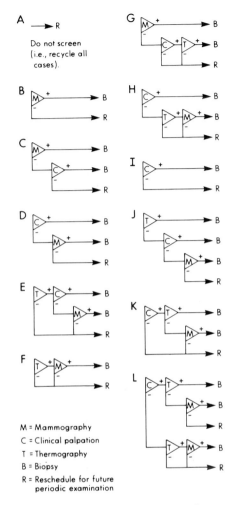

Fig. 8.12. Strategies appearing on expected cost surfaces.

tion. (See Fig. 8.12 for the precise definition of strategy *H* and all other strategies depicted in Fig. 8.6 to 8.11.)

Fig. 8.11 shows costs and regions of optimal strategies under the same conditions as in Fig. 8.10 except mammography is assigned a cost of $240. The region for strategy *D* has now been pushed back substantially by the new strategy *H*. Several new strategies, *I, J, K,* and *L,* appear over small regions because the high cost of mammography works against its use.

DISCUSSION

In the previous section the pattern of results was presented from the perspective of optimality. Only occasionally were suboptimal results mentioned. It is clear, however, that less-than-optimal strategies may be advantageous if at a slight increase in cost they are more natural to clinical practice or simpler to use. It has already been pointed out that strategies *C* and *D* are nearly the same in cost and that in fact only a slight increase in cost would result from always performing both a physical examination and mammography (which technically is dominated by both *C* and *D*).

Three-dimensional plots like Figs. 8.6 to 8.11 can be used effectively to judge whether one strategy can be extended into the region of another with only a small cost increase. Wherever a surface crease is hard to detect, the implication is that the two optimal strategies meeting there have almost identically sloping cost surfaces and can for all practical purposes be substituted for each other. For example, the strategies of the narrow regions in Figs. 8.10 and 8.11 can be replaced by adjacent strategies making *A, B, H,* and a variation of *D* or *C*, in which both mammography and clinical examination are done and biopsy is recommended if either is positive, the only strategies to be considered in practice.

One factor not considered in the discussion so far is the accuracy with which mammography is practiced. The implications of accuracy for examination frequency are substantial, as pointed out in Chapter 9. They are substantial in strategy selection also. Sensitivity and specificity rates for mammography at BCDDP No. 25 are as good as one can expect in most screening settings owing to 100 percent case follow-up and retrospective critique of mammograms for both cases missed and negative biopsy cases. The reviews were conducted by the mammographer who read all mammograms, working with the BCDDP coordinator.

Mammography would not play the major role described above in clinical settings where sensitivity and specificity rates are not as high as the rates from BCDDP No. 25 used in this analysis, namely, $TP \geq 58$ percent, $TN \geq 99$ percent. In such practices clinical palpation would probably be the modality of first choice with mammography used as a back-up modality, and early detection of a substantial fraction of breast cancers would not occur, thereby practically removing the potential advantages of early detection.

NOTES

1. In principle one could repeat the application of the same modalities indefinitely. In practice this is not an option unless, for example, an X-ray or thermographic image is unreadable. Then the test would be repeated during the same examination sequence and the new image(s) substituted for the inferior one(s). With this exclusion, retesting with the same modalities during the same examination sequence provides no new information, so that each test modality is applied no more than once.

2. But when independence is not maintained, the number of possible strategies is smaller from the outset.

3. As a point of departure we used $2 million as the expected value of an early, unnecessary death. Thus, per breast, the expected cost of a rad of radiation is on the order of (2×10^6)

$(6 \times 10^{-6}$ cancers yr^{-1} $rad^{-1})$ 20 yr $\times$ 0.5 = 120 dollar equivalents. We began with this estimate and varied it extensively to test the sensitivity of protocol selection to the estimate. Results are reported parametrically.

4. Sensitivity and specificity rates vary significantly for these three groups as illustrated in Chapter 7. And, of course, incidence rates increase with age.

5. Positive clinical examination refers to detection of a stellate or spiculated mass, especially if fixed to the skin or chest wall. Positive mammography refers to detection of one or more of the following features on the X-ray image: stellate or spiculated mass(es), a mass with ill-defined edges, scattered or clustered punctate calcifications, or localized architectural distortions of the breast. Less serious findings should be monitored for possible development but not biopsied for maximum detection accuracy. (See Chapter 7.)

REFERENCES

Boice JD, Land CE, Shore RE, Norman JE, Tokunaga M (1979) Risk of breast cancer following low-dose radiation exposure. Diagnostic Radiology 131: 589–597.

Bunker JP, Forrest WH, Mosteller, F, Vandam LD (1969) The National Halothane Study. Bethesda, Md., National Institutes of Health, USDHEW.

Gohagan, JK (1980) Quantitative analysis for public policy. New York, McGraw-Hill, Chap. 21.

Gohagan JK, Rodes ND, Blackwell CW, Darby WP, Farrell C, Herder T, Pearson DK, Spitznagel EL, Wallace MD (1980) Individual and combined effectiveness of palpation, thermography, and mammography in breast cancer screening. Preventive Medicine 9:713–721.

Mosteller F (1968) Association and estimation in contingency tables. Stat Assn 63:1–28.

United Nations Scientific Committee on Effects of Atomic Radiation (UNSCEAR) (1976) Radiation carcinogenesis in man. A/AC, 32/R.334. New York, United Nations.

Upton AC, Beebe GW, Brown JM, et al. (1977) Report of the NCI Ad Hoc Working Group on the risks associated with mammography in screening for the detection of breast cancer. J Nat Cancer Inst 59:481–493.

9

Risk-Benefit Trade-Off Considerations for Mammography: Examination Schedules

John K. Gohagan
William P. Darby

Mammography is superior to clinical palpation and other currently operational techniques for early detection of breast cancer [Gohagan et al. 1980a, 1980b]. This is a firm conclusion from our analysis, as documented in previous chapters. And there is plenty of evidence that this observation is true under a fairly wide range of conditions. For example, it was clearly demonstrated for women over 50 years of age in the New York Health Insurance Plan (HIP) study of the 1960s where 33 percent of the cancers were detected on mammography alone and the life expectancy for screened women was significantly greater than for unscreened controls with a 44 percent reduction in death from breast cancer after six years [Shapiro et al. 1974, Venet et al. 1971]. Furthermore, in the first year of the 27 Breast Cancer Detection Demonstration Projects (BCDDPs), an average of 44 percent of the cancers discovered were detected by mammography alone; because mammography is sensitive to smaller lesions, a large fraction, 33 percent, of the tumors detected were less than 1 cm in diameter, which bodes well for life expectancy [Beahrs et al. 1979, Gold 1978, Seidman 1977, Shapiro 1977, Shapiro et al. 1976].

On the other hand, mammography cannot be assumed to be risk free because X-radiation is carcinogenic even at low-dose levels, according to the best available scientific evidence. The United Nations Scientific Committee on Effects of Atomic Radiation critiqued the scientific literature on radiation carcinogenesis in man and concluded that X-radiation as low as 1 rad, approximately the dosage of a Xerox mammographic examination, could generate cancers at the rate of 3.5 to 7.5 per year per million population exposed beginning 10 years after exposure and continuing for life [McGregor et al. 1977, UNSCEAR 1976]. More recent studies confirm the inherent riskiness of X-radiation [Boice et al. 1979, Morgan 1979, Upton et al. 1977].

Although this tension between benefits and risks is widely appreciated, the magnitude of the risk associated with occasional and regular mammography cannot be precisely calculated. Certainly BCDDP data are inadequate for the task. The best per-rad estimates of risk are those mentioned above. But even with this limitation, the risk-benefit trade-off relation has not been adequately characterized in the medical literature for authoritative clinical decision making. In this chapter we present an equation for estimating lifetime risk as a function of the number, frequency, and timing of mammographic examinations. The equation includes age-specific mortality rates as a means of depleting the at-risk population with age. We use this equation to calculate the lifetime risk for a number of realistic scenarios incorporating repeated mammograms. Then we apply decision analysis techniques to determine the conditions under which the expected benefits of a mammographic examination for early detection of breast cancer at a particular point in a woman's life outweigh the risks. The conditions are specified in terms of the accuracy of mammography in clinical settings; the costs of detection, diagnosis, and treatment; and the statistical chance that a woman at a specific age with a specified family and medical history, including previous X rays, is likely to be harboring a cancer. It is not possible to specify a single optimal lifetime protocol for mammography for all women, but we do demonstrate appropriate protocols for average and high-risk women using the best current estimates of radiation risk and a wide range of realistic cost factors. Finally, we explain the cost and risk implications of the current American Cancer Society (ACS) policy on screening asymptomatic women using mammography.

RISK ESTIMATION

In the medical and epidemiological literature the term *risk* is used variously to mean the lifetime probability of contracting a disease, the probability that a disease is present at a given point in time (prevalence), and the probability of developing a disease in a specified time interval (incidence).

The annual risk of developing breast cancer as a result of X-ray mammography is dependent upon the midbreast average dose of radiation received [Boice et al. 1979, Upton et al. 1977]. The per-rad risk of low-dose mammography has not been determined experimentally. Instead, estimates have been made by extrapolation from high-dose situations. The best current estimate of carcinogenic risk from X-radiation are those given above [Upton et al. 1977]. They derive from the assumption that the curve relating dose to tumor incidence may be linear or nonlinear in the low-dose region of less than 50 rads where empirical data are not available for curve fitting [NCRP 1980]. See Fig. 9.1.

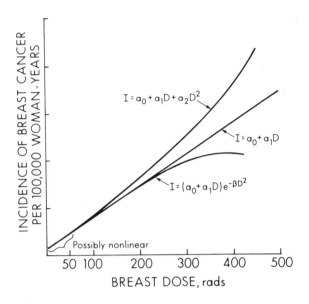

I = Incidence
D = Dose, in rads
β = A parameter to capture possible cell-killing effects at high doses
a_0, a_1, a_2 are constants

FIG. 9.1. Models for extrapolating low-dose risk from high-dose risk data. The linear fit has been shown to be adequate [NCRP 1980].

In the 1960s a complete mammogram exposed a woman to 7 to 15 rads per breast [Feig 1979]. Improved techniques, including the use of intensifying screens in film cassettes, have made high-resolution mammography practical with less than 1 rad of midbreast exposure [Feig 1979, Gold 1978, Jaeger 1975]. Under controlled circumstances dose levels of less than 0.5 rad per examination have been achieved. Dose levels associated with mammography in clinical settings range from 0.06 rad at midbreast per craniocaudal view (0.12 rad per two-view examination) for film/screen systems with a tungsten anode to more than 1 rad for a direct film exposure system. Average doses nationwide are 0.16 rad per examination for film/screen systems, 0.6 rad for Xerox mammography, and 0.82 rad for direct film exposure [Gold 1978, Jans and Ohlhaber 1979, Jensen and Butler 1978].

With these estimates plus the age-specific survivorship function for women for all diseases and a survivorship relation for the women in whom radiogenesis of breast tumors occurs, the number of cancers per million women exposed is easily estimated according to the equation below, assuming one exposure:

$$N = \alpha\beta (P_{t+10} + P_{t+11} + \ldots + P_{t+30})$$

In this equation N is the expected number of cancers due to an examination in year t, and α is the number of cancers generated per rad of exposure per million women per year for life after 10 years ($3.5 \leq \alpha \leq 7.5$) [Upton et al. 1977].

Table 9.1 shows the results of computerized tabulation of the total number of cancers generated for numerous reasonable scenarios. For periodic exposures over time the expression for N is modified to account for accumulating annual risk. For example, the number of cancers expected between ages 50 and 70 years from a series of 10 annual mammograms beginning at age 40 years is

$$N = \alpha\beta (P_{t+10} + 2P_{t+11} + \ldots + 2OP_{t+30})$$

where t is the age at which the first mammogram is done, and the numerical multipliers account for annual accumulations of risk for exposures 10 or more years previous. α is the carcinogenesis rate as defined above, and β is the probability of surviving the breast cancer if one is generated ($\beta \cong 0.5$) [Morgan 1979]. P_{t+i} is the probability of living i years after the X-ray exposure; it is the survivorship function for women in the risk group for all diseases other than a radiogenerated breast cancer [U.S. NCHS 1978].[1]

The number of additional cancers to a population of mammographed women can be fairly large, larger than one might suspect. And when contrasted with national standards for chemical carcinogens, their magnitudes loom enormous. For example, some regulatory agencies consider unreasonable an increased lifetime risk of 100 cancers per million people exposed to saccharin, trihalomethanes in drinking water, or vinyl chloride in the workplace. Yet repeated irradiation of the breasts can easily generate more cancers according to current risk data. One might be inclined to discount

TABLE 9.1.
Cumulative Additional Cancers Expected for an Initial Population
of 1 Million White Women Subjected to Appropriate National Mortality Rates

	Per-Rad Carcinogenesis Rate			
	Cancers per Million Women per Year after 10 Years			
Exposure scenario	1.0	3.5	6.0	7.5
1 rad at age 30	35	124	212	266
1 rad at age 20	45	158	271	338
1 rad every 10 years from age 30	86	302	518	647
1 rad each year from age 50	178	623	1,069	1,336
1 rad every 2 years from age 30	356	1,246	2,137	2,671
1 rad each year from age 40	389	1,363	2,337	2,921

radiation risk from mammography by observing that exposure to 1 rad of ionizing radiation at age 30 years increases lifetime risk only by about 124 to 266 cancers per million women, or to about a 7.02 percent lifetime chance of breast cancer (using the usually quoted 7 percent as the national average lifetime risk in the absence of radiogenesis). Even annual mammograms from age 40 years on increases risk to at most 7.3 percent. However, by ignoring radiation risk one ignores the reality that the women in whom these cancers are induced would not have developed the disease at all in the absence of the radiation exposure. For these women the consequences are severe. On the other hand, the benefits to women in whom cancer is discovered early can be significant.[2] Since a woman can never know for certain the probability of her being in one group or the other, she must consider both sides of the issue in deciding for or against mammography, as discussed in the next section.

RISK-BENEFIT DECISION MODEL

Decisions regarding the use of mammography depend on striking a rational balance between increased risk and anticipated benefits. Clinicians are here faced with a classic situation where a potentially beneficial course of action carries with it the possibility of a substantial negative consequence with a low probability. The natural human tendency is to discount highly improbable outcomes as being essentially impossible. But decision analysts have shown that the wiser thing to do is to consider both the probability and the magnitude of all consequences explicitly as a basis for choice [Raiffa 1968]. The proper framework for problems of this type is the paradigm of formal decision analysis in which the alternatives are compared on the basis of expected utility when utility functions can be assessed and on the basis of expected net benefit or expected net cost when they cannot; we are restricted in our analysis to the objective of minimizing expected cost since assessments of utility functions are practically out of the question.

The decision tree in Fig. 9.2 characterizes the decision problem faced by a woman and her physician considering the alternatives of doing a mammogram in a particular instance. Without knowing for certain whether breast cancer is present, the choice must be made and the consequences (the financial and psychosocial costs) of the chosen action incurred. Each branch of the decision tree represents a different outcome situation.

The number P_c is the probability that cancer is present. It is estimated approximately using national age-specific prevalence and incidence data for breast cancer modified to reflect the presence of important risk features. The only risk-modifying features so employed are age and previous history of breast X rays. We cannot make further modifications with any confidence to reflect other epidemiological features, such as age at menarche and reproductive history, because convincing, scientifically valid,

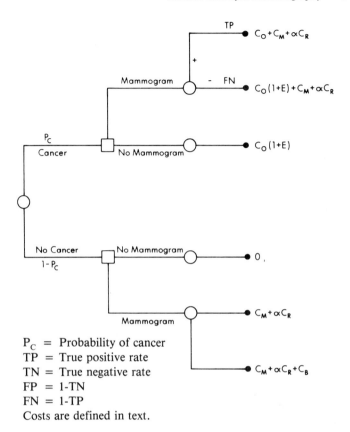

P_C = Probability of cancer
TP = True positive rate
TN = True negative rate
FP = 1-TN
FN = 1-TP
Costs are defined in text.

FIG. 9.2. Simplified decision tree for periodic mammograms.

multivariate risk studies on these features appear not to have been done yet.[3] (See Chapter 6.)

The other probabilities on the tree reflect the combined capabilities of the technology and the interpreter of the mammogram. They are the probability of a positive examination when cancer is present, the true positive (*TP*) rate for mammography, the probability of a positive examination when cancer is absent, the false positive (*FP*) rate, and two complementary probabilities, namely, the false negative rate, $FN = 1 - TP$, and the true negative rate, $TN = 1 - FP$. These probabilities might be called calibration probabilities for mammography, for, as discussed in Chapter 7, they measure the capability of the technology to distinguish between cancerous and noncancerous breasts. In principle they can be measured for any clinical setting. In practice we cannot know their precise values in most clinical settings because sufficient data do not exist, but we do know their approximate values from data for BCDDP No. 25 and from rates reported for other BCDDPs [Beahrs et al. 1979, Gohagan et al. 1980a, Hicks 1979].

Only costs are shown for outcomes. The possible benefits from early detection are incorporated in terms of lower costs of treatment. Treatment costs are quite complex and vary by extent of disease and procedure. Average treatment costs are used as the starting point of analysis, and the sensitivity to cost values are investigated in the analysis.[4] The specific costs included are

C_O—average cost of treatment for cancers detected early, losses in earning power that might occur subsequent to detection of a breast cancer, and possible psychosocial costs.

C_M—cost of doing a mammogram.

C_R—average cost of cancers generated by mammography. In financial terms this would mean treatment cost, but psychosocial costs are even higher.

n—lifetime probability of a cancer due to the mammogram. This is numerically equal to 10^{-6} times the N previously calculated. This number times the average cost of mammography-generated cancers is the expected long-term cost of the radiation.

C_B—cost of a biopsy.

k—a multipier to account for the fact that cancers that are missed on an early examination have a good chance of metastisizing before they are eventually detected, thereby requiring more costly treatment and leading to a less positive (more costly) prognosis. The value of this multiplier probably declines slowly with age beyond some point because economic opportunity costs decline and the competition for a life intensifies with age [Gohagan and Swift, 1981]. Financial data for the analysis are from Washington University Medical Center and published data from national studies. (See Appendix B.) Psychosocial costs cannot be estimated accurately and are treated parametrically. Similarly, the multiplier k is treated as a parameter for variation in sensitivity analysis.

Evaluation of the decision tree of Fig. 9.2 is straightforward. The objective is to determine the minimum probability P_C for which the use of mammography provides sufficient benefit to offset its risks.[5] First, the expected cost of mammography is calculated when cancer is present, $E(M/Ca)$. Then the expected cost of mammography is calculated when cancer is absent, $E(M/\overline{Ca})$[6]. These two expected costs are weighed by the probabilities P_C and $1 - P_C$, respectively, to find the overall expected cost of the decision to use mammography in an arbitrary case $E(M)$. The calculations yield

$$E(M/Ca) = C_O + C_M + nC_R + FNkC_O$$
$$E(M/\overline{Ca}) = FPC_B + C_M + nC_R$$
$$E(M) = P_C E(M/Ca) + (1 - P_C) E(M/\overline{Ca})$$
$$= C_M + nC_R + P_C(C_O + FNkC_O - FPC_B) + FPC_B$$

Next the expected value of not using mammography is calculated in similar fashion:

$$E(\bar{M}) = P_c E(\bar{M}/Ca) + (1 - P_c) E(\bar{M}/\overline{Ca})$$
$$= P_c C_o (1 + k)$$

The best of the two options, whether to apply mammography at the time in question, is the one with the lowest expected cost. That is, mammography is warranted only if $E(M) < E(\bar{M})$. Substituting the previously calculated expected costs, $E(M)$ and $E(\bar{M})$, into this condition and solving for P_c yields the practical decision rule that mammography is warranted only if P_c is larger than a threshold ratio incorporating the costs and probabilities associated with a specific situation. The ratio has the form

$$P_c > \frac{(C_M + nC_R + FPC_B)}{(C_o kTP + FPC_B)}$$

This threshold ratio is quite sensitive to the calibration probabilities *TP* and *FP* and to C_o and k. It is not very sensitive to the per-rad carcinogenic rate α. Within the 3.5 to 7.5 range the only effect is that larger α values lead to more frequent recommendations for mammography among women in their seventies to help detect possible radiogenerated cancers induced by repeated screening earlier in their lives. Setting α to 0.5 results in essentially the same screening schedules as for α equal to 3.5. Nor is the ratio very sensitive to the financial costs for mammography and biopsy within the ranges of uncertainty in our estimates. The relationship of the threshold ratio to prevalence and incidence is shown in Fig. 9.3 for various

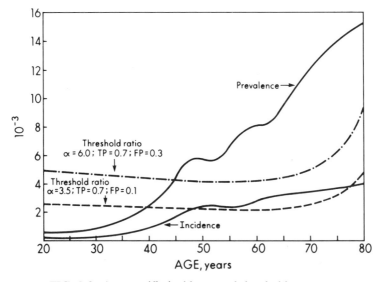

FIG. 9.3. Age-specific incidence and threshold curves.

values of *TP*, *FP*, and α. The effect of *k* is evident in the upward curving tails of the threshold ratio as *k* declines slowly toward zero beyond age 50 years.

Table 9.2 depicts a few representative lifetime protocols derived from the analysis. They are based on year-by-year applications of the inequality above. Each year, P_c is recalculated based on age and previous X-ray history before comparing it with the threshold ratio; X rays done a decade or more previously contribute at a fixed annual rate to overall risk for surviving women. Mammography is employed first in the year in which the prevalence rate initially exceeds the threshold ratio. It is next repeated for an asymptomatic woman (no physical evidence of the disease) when her accumulated risk calculated from total statistical incidence for the intervening period, including cancers missed and the accumulated risk from previous X rays, exceeds the threshold ratio.[7]

DISCUSSION

The three most important considerations in the decision to recommend a mammogram are accuracy of the technique in the clinical setting (in terms of true positive and false positive rates), the relative magnitudes of the costs associated with earlier versus later detection of cancers, and the woman's inherent epidemiological risk level, P_c, at the time of decision. There is also a limited trade-off relation between radiation dose per examination and test accuracy, as one would expect, which provides a rationale for doing not-so-accurate low-dose mammography more often than one could justify similarly inaccurate higher-dose exams. However, this is a weak relation that is dominated by the other factors and should not contribute except secondarily to scheduling decisions.

True positive rates as low as 50 percent and false positive rates as high as 10 percent to 30 percent for mammography are not uncommon in the literature [Menitoff 1978]. BCDDP number 23 reported true and false positive rates of 0.6 and 0.5, respectively [Hicks et al. 1979]. Clinics operating at such low-accuracy rates should use mammography sparingly even among high-risk asymptomatic women because the frequencies of unnecessary biopsy and of missed cancers are high and the balance of benefits to risk is not favorable. Only when the perceived costs of a cancer missed are exceedingly high, many hundreds of thousands of dollars in financial and psychosocial costs, is mammography appropriate in these low-accuracy settings.

If, on the other hand, a clinic has empirically established mammographic accuracy rates of $TP = 55$ percent to 60 percent and $FP = 1$ percent to 2 percent or better, our analysis shows that annual mammograms are desirable for high-risk (average $+20\text{–}50\%$) women in the sixth decade, with triennial mammograms between the ages of 42 and 47 years and bien-

TABLE 9.2.

Appropriate Mammographic Sequences for White U.S. Women, Assuming 1 Rad at Midbreast per Two-View Mammogram

Treatment and Psychosocial Cost Detection Early	Treatment and Psychosocial Cost Metastatic	Nonradiological Relative Risk	True Positive and False Positive Rates	Cancers Generated for Per-Rad Risk of			Cancers Detected
				3.5	6.0	7.5	
5,000	50,000	Avg + 20%	$TP = 0.58$; $FP = 0.02$[a]	384	659	824	51,599
5,000	25,000	Avg	x x x x x x x xxxxxxxxxxxxxxxxx x x x	147	252	313	40,498
			xx x xxxxxxxxxxx x x x x x x x				
5,000	50,000	Avg + 20%	$TP = 0.82$; $FP = 0.02$[b]	603	1,033	1,291	82,350
5,000	25,000	Avg	x x x xxxxxxxxxxxxxxxxxxxxxxxxxxxxx x x	249	427	533	63,373
			x xxxxxxxxxxxxxxx x x x x x				
1,000 to 10,000	100,000	Avg + 50%	$TP = 0.6$; $FP = 0.5$[c]	268	459	575	71,093
1,000 to 10,000	100,000	Avg	x xxxxxxxxxxxxxxxxxxx x	166	284	355	42,853
1,000 to 10,000	100,000	Avg − 20%	x x x x x x x x x x x x x	69	119	148	24,166
			x x x x x x x x				
			40 age (in years) 80				

[a]Rates for BCDDP No. 25 mammographer.

[b]Rates for BCDDP No. 25 with clinical palpation and mammography done sequentially but independently.

[c]Rates for the Arizona BCDDP mammographers [Hicks et al. 1979].

Note: The following costs were assumed, but the results are insensitive to variations of ± 20 percent: mammogram, $50; biopsy, $600; psychosocial costs were dealt with parametrically. Cost for radiation risk is not included. At 10 years 50 percent survival was presumed. Calculations incorporate standard U.S. life tables. Schedules do not change, but cancers generated scale linearly with midbreast dose. Schedules do change with increased costs for metastatic cancers. Cancers are per million women examined.

nial mammograms otherwise. In these high-accuracy clinics biennial mammograms are optimal for women of average risk after 45 years with annual mammograms between the ages of 50 and 70 years.

The reason for continuing X-ray examinations well into the seventies or even into the eighties is the increased risk from previous X rays. In the absence of previous X rays incidence rates fall off enough in the sixth decade for women of average risk to discontinue the periodic mammogram in favor of clinical palpation. For $\alpha \leq 3.5$ mammography typically can be discontinued after about age 70 years, whereas for $\alpha \geq 7.5$ enough new cancers are generated to warrant continuing the test regularly through the seventies.

Although our results are couched in terms of relative risk level, we have not found a sound scientific basis for classifying asymptomatic women with no previous disease as below or above average risk beyond accounting for age and previous X-ray history, as pointed out in earlier chapters. On the other hand, we have no basis for completely ignoring the concepts of low and high risk. The risk ranges we used in our analysis, average to 100 percent above average, are modest in comparison to some values reported in the literature. But upon analysis of BCDDP data and critique of the methods and data used by authors quoting much higher risk, we judge this to be an adequate range.

In the discussion so far we have not addressed the question of whether mammography should be used alone or in concert with clinical palpation. It is standard practice to couple mammography with clinical palpation of the breasts, and in Chapter 8 we demonstrated that this two-modality strategy is, though not optimal in all cases, at least a close runner-up to the optimal strategy. Our analysis in the current chapter holds whether one assumes this standard practice or assumes instead that mammography is being considered as a solo procedure, so long as the true positive and true negative rates for the protocol used (mammography alone or with clinical palpation) are within the ranges discussed. However, one can expect higher true positive rates with little reduction in true negative rates with the two-modality protocol. More frequent screening would then be appropriate. For example, BCDDP No. 25 achieved true positive and true negative rates for mammography of 58 percent and 98 percent respectively, leading us to recommend an optimal schedule of biennial mammograms after 45 years and annual mammograms between 50 and 70 years of age for asymptomatic women. But when screening with mammography and clinical palpation (each done independently), BCDDP No. 25 achieved rates of 82 percent and 98 percent, a vast improvement due to the complementarity of the two modalities. With those exceptionally high rates annual screening after age 45 years is optimal.

Because so many factors should legitimately influence decisions regarding mammography, those responsible for recommending a course of actions should carefully weigh the costs and probabilities, as we have shown, for their own situations. From the clinician's perspective the costs to be weighed should reflect the perspective of the patient and should include opportunity costs such as wages and other income foregone as well as test costs paid for out of pocket but not costs borne by other parties. And psychological trauma of induced cancers, of cancers overlooked, and of negative biopsies should be reflected in the cost magnitudes to give a better perspective.

In most clinical settings direct calculation of the threshold ratio may be practically impossible. We recommend, therefore, that clinicians match accuracy rates for their practices to those portrayed in Table 9.2 and adopt a protocol that approximately matches one of those for which treatment costs are between $1,000 and $10,000. (True and false positive rates for individual clinics should be established by proper methods of data collection and statistical analysis over a reasonable time period; a good statistician should lead the effort.) Until clinic-specific rates are established, most clinics should assume rates substantially less accurate than $TP = 0.6$ and $FP = 0.1$ for mammography alone and 0.82 and 0.1 for clinical palpation and mammography in combination. These are appropriate only for clinics where mammography is a speciality and interpretation is meticulously monitored for accuracy via patient follow-up (both positive and negative cases).

We close with a comment. From the analysis and discussion above we must conclude that the 1980 ACS policy on screening for breast cancer using clinical examination and mammography (annual examinations beginning in the mid-to-late forties) implicitly assumes very high accuracy rates for mammography in the average clinical setting. We find no evidence in the literature to justify such an assumption. We doubt that the average clinic achieves sufficiently high accuracy rates to justify annual mammograms for asymptomatic women. Biennial mammograms would probably be more appropriate in most clinical settings.

NOTES

1. The data were corrected for deaths due to breast cancer using incidence data and survivor data for the disease.

2. There is not a one-to-one trade-off between cancers generated and cancers detected. Individuals do not view these possibilities as balanced. These issues are illustrated effectively in Weinstein and Feinberg [1980].

3. Current suspicious physical features such as skin changes, architectural distortion, and nipple discharges are not considered because these are features of the disease that are evident even on physical palpation and cannot therefore be considered risk features for early detection by mammography. If any of these features are present, P_c is high enough that mammography is appropriate.

4. Sensitivity analysis is absolutely essential in studies where parameters cannot be

precisely calculated. Only in this way can one determine the parametric bounds within which one decision alternative is superior to another. For this reason we investigated the decision implication of all parameters of the model in the course of analysis. All important results are reported in the text.

5. Keep in mind that benefits are incorporated as negative costs, or cost savings.

6. A bar over a symbol means "not." For example, $\overline{Ca}$ means cancer is not present, and $\overline{M}$ means mammography is not done.

7. The incidence data used in the analysis are empirical annual rates reported for the BCDDPs. The rates each year reflect a mix of newly detectable cancers plus more-advanced cancers missed in the previous year.

REFERENCES

Beahrs, OH, Shapiro S, Smart C, et al. (1979) Report of the Working Group to Review the NCI/ACS Breast Cancer Detection Demonstration Projects. J Natl Cancer Inst 62:641–709.

Boice JD, Land CE, Shore RE, Norman JE, Tokunaga M (1979) Risk of breast cancer following low-dose radiation exposure. Diagnostic Radiology 131:589–597.

Feig SA (1979) Hypothetical breast cancer risk from mammography: a reassuring assessment. Breast: Diseases of the Breast 5:2–6.

Gohagan JK (1980) Quantitative analysis for public policy. New York, McGraw-Hill, chaps. 18–21.

Gohagan JK, Rodes ND, Blackwell CW, Darby WP, Farrell C, Herder T, Pearson DK, Spitznagel EL, Wallace MD (1980a) Individual and combined effectiveness of palpation, thermography, and mammography in breast cancer screening. Preventive Medicine 9:713–721.

Gohagan JK, Rodes ND, et al. (1980b) Screening for breast cancer: mammography is superior to clinical palpation. Letter to the editor. New Engl J Med 32:60.

Gohagan JK, Swift JG (1981) Scheduling Pap smears for asymptomatic women. Preventive Medicine 10:741–753.

Gold RH (1978) Mammography: is it worth the risk? Who should have mammography and when? UCLA Cancer Bulletin 5:3–7.

Hicks MJ, Davis JR, Layton JM, Present AJ (1979) Sensitivity of mammography and physical examination of the breast for detecting breast cancer. JAMA 242:2080–2083.

Jaeger SS, Cacak RK, Barnes JE, et al. (1975) Optimizing of Xeroradiographic exposures. Radiology 128:217–222.

Jans RG, Butler PF, McCrohan JL, Jr., Thompson WE (1979) The status of film/screen mammography. Radiology 132:197–200.

Jans RG, Ohlhaber TR (1979) Reduced dose mammography . . . results of a nationwide study, in Logan WW and Muntz EP (eds), Reduced dose mammography. New York, Masson.

Jensen JE, Butler PF (1978) Breast exposure: nationwide trends; mammographic quality assurance program results to date. Radiologic Technology 50:251–257.

McGregor DH, Land CE, Choc K, et al. (1977) Breast cancer incidence among atomic bomb survivors, Hiroshima and Nagasaki, 1950–1969. J Natl Cancer Inst 59:799–811.

Menitoff R (1978) A decision analytic approach to the evaluation of alternative breast cancer screening practices and strategies. Masters thesis. Sever Institute of Technology, School of Engineering and Applied Science, Washington University, St. Louis, Mo.

Morgan R (1979) Benefit-risk ratios in mammography. Presented as acceptance speech upon receiving the Roentgen Medal in the Roentgen Museum, W. Germany, 14 May. Referenced with permission.

National Council on Radiation Protection and Measurements (1980) Mammography Recommendations of the National Council on Radiation Protection and Measurements, NCRP no. 66. Washington, D.C. NCRP.

United Nations Scientific Committee on Effects of Atomic Radiation (UNSCEAR) (1976) Radiation Carcinogenesis in Man. A/AC, 32/R.334. New York: United Nations.

Raiffa H (1968) Decision analysis: introductory lectures on choices under uncertainty. Reading, Mass., Addison Wesley.

Seidman H (1977) Screening for breast cancer in younger women, life expectancy gains and losses: an analysis according to risk indicator groups. CA 27:66–87.

Shapiro S (1977) Evidence on screening for breast cancer from a randomized trial. Cancer 39:2772–2782.

Shapiro S, Strax P, Venet L (1976) Evaluation of periodic breast cancer screening with mammography: methodology and early observations. JAMA 195:111–118.

Shapiro S, Strax P, Venet L, Venet W (1974) Changes in 5-year breast cancer mortality in a breast cancer screening program, *in* Seventh National Cancer Conference Proceedings, pp. 663–678. Washington, D.C., American Cancer Society, January 1974.

U.S., National Center for Health Statistics (1978) Vital statistics of the United States. Washington, D.C.: Government Printing Office.

Upton AC, Beebe GW, Brown JM, et al. (1977) Report of NCI Ad Hoc Working Group on the risks associated with mammography in screening for the detection of breast cancer. J Natl Cancer Inst 59:481–493.

Venet L, Strax P, Venet W, Shapiro S (1971) Adequacies and inadequacies of breast examination by physicians in mass screening. Cancer 28:1546–1550.

Weinstein MC, Feinberg HV (1980) Clinical decision analysis. Philadelphia, W. B. Saunders, chaps. 3, 7.

PART III

Summary of Results and Therapeutic Implications

Chapter 10 summarizes the clinically relevant aspects of Part I and Part II. It is not a substitute for the earlier chapters, but it does cover the major conclusions. Chapter 11 provides an overview of current surgical procedures and other treatment modalities for breast cancer and provides some insight into the therapeutic value of early detection. While one can not be certain that early detection will yield improved therapeutic results in any specific case, increased longevity, at least for older women, was demonstrated statistically by the controlled clinical trial conducted by the New York Health Insurance Plan. Also, less severe therapeutic procedures are applicable in many cases of premetastatic (early-detected) breast cancer.

10

Summary of Results

John K. Gohagan

This chapter highlights the clinically relevant findings of our study and important related facts from the literature. The reader should keep clearly in mind that the discussion here and elsewhere in this work pertains to asymptomatic women only. Results from analyses of data from Breast Cancer Detection Demonstration Project (BCDDP) No. 25 and results that derive from mathematical modeling and the use of data from other sources are distinguished.

PATIENT RISK ASSESSMENT

A variety of epidemiological and medical features have beem implicated as risk modifiers in the published literature. Those features commonly believed to be important for classifying asymptomatic women as high, low, or average risk were summarized in Chapter 6. BCDDP No. 25 collected data in the form of medical histories for all 10,187 women screened reflecting the presence and scale of these features.

Univariate comparisons of feature occurrences among participants who developed cancer and those who did not would appear to confirm the importance of many of these features as risk modifiers. However, univariate comparisons can be misleading and are inappropriate for risk assessments of women with two or more possibly interrelated features such as age and the use of birth control pills. Multivariate discriminant analyses of these data, controlling for age, lead us to hypothesize that the really imporant risk feature is age. A family history of breast cancer may be a second important feature; although BCDDP No. 25 data seem to suggest this relationship, there are too few women in the project whose mothers, grand-mothers, aunts, or sisters had breast cancer to provide valid statistical support for such a conclusion. The other suspected risk features are con-founded by age and do not contribute significantly to risk as independent variables. Since other researchers have typically not controlled for age or other confounding features in their studies, preferring to make univariate in lieu of multivariate comparisons, we are reluctant to accept results from published studies that are at variance with ours. The one study that we know did control for age appears to be in agreement with the conclusion [Egan et al. 1977].

Again, BCDDP No. 25 data cannot be used to test directly the hypothesis that the number of previous breast X rays is a modifier of risk. However, the potential hazard from X rays has been shown from biological studies and large-scale international epidemiological studies on the risks of ionizing radiation. The magnitude of risk is not certain, but the best scien-tific estimates at this time are 3.5 to 7.5 additional cancers per year generated per million women exposed to a rad of radiation at midbreast be-ginning 10 years after exposure and continuing for life [Boice et al. 1979, UNSCEAR 1977, Upton et al. 1977].

Our conclusions on risk features are summarized in Table 10.1.

TEST MODALITY INTERPRETATION

The three detection modalities employed at BCDDP No. 25 were clinical palpation and visual inspection of the breasts and the associated lymph system, Xerox mammography, and thermography, as described in Chapters 3 and 4. These tests were done independently. Specifically, 14 basic features were examined for via clinical palpation and inspection, 21 via mammography, and 4 via thermography. The best predictors of malig-nant disease are listed for clinical examination and mammography in Table 10.2. The chance that a malignancy is present in an asymptomatic woman is substantially increased when features from either of these two groupings are observed. The other features included in our evaluations were not good predictors of malignancy. None of the thermographic features were statistically significant predictors of disease either individually or in groups. (See Chapter 7.)

True positive rates (sensitivity) and true negative rates (specificity) for the three individual modalities and mixed-modality protocols are given in Table 10.3[1] They were calculated using only data from those examinations in the first four years where all three tests were done. This ensured com-parability of results and sufficient time in the fifth year of the project to determine the true status of women at the time of their fourth-year ex-amination using pathology reports and follow-up. For Xerox mam-mography the overall true positive rate was about 58 percent and the true

TABLE 10.1
Conclusions on Epidemiological Risk Features.

| Variable | Data Source | |
	BCDDP No. 25	Literature
Family history with other cancers	Not significant	Not convincing
Late first childbirth	Not significant	Not convincing
One child or less	Not significant	Not convincing
Limited or no breast feeding	Not significant	Not convincing
Early menarche or late menopause	Not significant	Not convincing
Age	Risk increases significantly with age	Risk increases significantly with age
Family history with breast cancer	Insufficient data	Probably risk influencing
Repeated breast X rays	No data	Magnitude of risk increase uncertain

Note: Based on review of literature and multivariate analysis of BCDDP No. 25 data.

negative rate was about 99 percent. For clinical examination and thermography the respective rates were about 26 percent and 99 percent versus 39 percent and 91 percent. In our judgment these rates reflect the level of sensitivity and specificity to be expected in screening programs. The three tests were done independently, which is essential for evaluation; individual examiners knew nothing of the results of the previous tests. Also the thermographer and the mammographer saw only the films, although the mam-

TABLE 10.2
Best Statistical Predictors of Malignancy with Mammography and Palpation.

Mammography (15 variables considered)
  Irregularly shaped mass—stellate, spiculated, multinodular, indistinct edges
  Clustered or punctate calcifications
  Localized architectual distortion, indeterminant density
  Localized skin thickening
Clinical palpation (10 variables considered)
  Irregularly shaped mass
  Mass fixed to skin or fixed deep
  Hard mass
  Unilateral nipple discharge, especially bloody
  Skin retraction
  Nipple retraction

Note: Order of listing indicates declining predictability within each group.

TABLE 10.3
Optimal True Positive and True Negative Rates for Protocols

Protocol	True Positive Rate*	True Negative Rate*
Mammography alone	53	98
Palpation alone	49	94
Palpation with mammography	59	98

*The true positive rate, the fraction of cancers detected by a test modality or protocol, is a statistical approximation to test sensitivity. The true negative rate, the fraction of no-cancer cases testing negative, is an approximation to test specificity.

Notes: These rates were calculated using logistic regression techniques. (See Chapter 7.) The features variables listed in Table 2.3 were included individually and in combinations. The rates given can be achieved on the average by recommending biopsy if any of the features listed are observed. Rates are significantly lower when other less important features like nipple discharge are used as a basis for recommending biopsy because of the nonspecificity of these features for breast cancer. Actual rates achieved are at variance with these, indicating that examiners had information beyond that recorded as features.

mographer used a previous X-ray film for comparison and knew the woman's age. The clinicians saw the women, of course, and did question them during the palpation.

Based on published studies, mammographic practice generally appears to fall short of its practical potential [Hicks et al. 1979, Menitoff 1977]. If radiologist interpreters were to focus on the image features listed in Table 10.2 and implement quality control procedures like those discussed below, the effectiveness of mammography in clinical practices might improve substantially. Sensitivity and specificity rates for mammogaphy at BCDDP No. 25 are potentially achievable in any clinical setting.[2]

When BCDDP No. 25 data were grouped by the presence or absence of lymph node involvement, an indication of metastatic cancer and larger tumors, the rates for mammography and thermography remained essentially unchanged; mammography was consistently sensitive and specific regardless of lymph node involvement, and thermography was relatively insensitive and unspecific. But clinical examination was found to be nearly as sensitive as mammography when lymph nodes were involved and much less sensitive, though more specific, than thermography in the absence of lymph node involvement [Gohagan et al. 1980].

Although mammography is clearly the best individual early detection technique, it is important to observe that mammography alone may not be the best protocol or strategy for early detection, depending on one's view of the relative importance of false positive and false negative examinations. In particular the use of both clinical examination and mammography with biopsy recommended if either is positive increases sensitivity substantially to about 82 percent while reducing specificity only one percentage point to 98 percent.

QUALITY CONTROL PRACTICES

Quality control is as important in medicine as in other human activities [Gohagan et al. 1981]. But, although it could be, it is seldom practiced in clinical settings to the extent that our analyses suggest it should. Both clinical examination and mammography were subjected to rigorous quality control procedures at BCDDP No. 25. And judging by the literature on test accuracy, these procedures had an observable impact on the effectiveness of those examination modalities.

The most important and underutilized element of quality control is case follow-up. A random sample of all cases found negative on examination should be followed for at least one year. Cancers detected within one year may well have been detectable at the time of the previous negative examination, and retrospective evaluation of those examination data, especially radiological images, can reveal subtle features missed in the original examination and provide the grist for refining feature interpretations. Reviews of negative examination data for subsequently developing cancer cases make possible a more precise allocation of cases into true and false negative categories for more accurate estimation and enhancement of sensitivity and specificity rates as can be seen from Table 10.4, which is a simplified version of cross-tabulated examination data in symbolic form.

All cases for which biopsy is recommended should be reviewed regularly in clinical settings doing only a few examinations per day to determine the true disease state at the time of examination and to provide additional insight especially into features that are not good predictors.[3] Here, too, review is important to a precise allocation of cases into true and false positive categories for accurate estimates of sensitivity and specificity.

TABLE 10.4
Illustrative Cross-tabulation for Sensitivity, Specificity,
and Predictive Value Calculations

Histology	Examination Results for Modality		
	Positive	**Negative**	**Total**
Cancer	A^a	B^b	$A + B$
No cancer	C^a	D^b	$C + D$
Total	$A + C$	$B + D$	$A + B + C + D$

TP (sensitivity) $= A/(A + B) = 1 - FN$.
TN (specificity) $= D/(C + D) = 1 - FP$.
Predictive value of positive exam $= A/(A + C)$.
[a]Lack of follow-up of negative biopsied cases leads to imprecise distributions of positively examined cases between A and C, thereby affecting sensitivity and specificity rates.
[b]Lack of follow-up of negative exam cases typically inflates D and deflates B, leading to possibly substantially inflated sensitivity plus mildly deflated specificity rates.

Clinics screening large numbers of women daily need review only a sample of cases.

Quality control should be the responsibility of individual examiners. Accuracy rates are bound to vary among examiners even for the same modality because of differences in experience, focus, and attention to detail. The overall quality of a clinic will reflect the capabilities of associated examiners and will improve as examiners both individually and as an information-sharing group enhance their performances.

RISK-BENEFIT BALANCE FOR MAMMOGRAPHY

The issue of risk-benefit balance for mammography is widely discussed in the literature [for example, Berlin 1978, Culliton 1977, Fox et al. 1978, Gold 1977]. But the analyses have not been done properly. More precisely, 3.5 to 7.5 new cancers per year per rad of exposure beginning after a 10-year latency period may seem tiny, as many authors argue. (See Chapters 8 and 9.) But each examination by Xerox mammography provides nearly 1 rad of radiation per breast at midline.[4] And annual exposures from 40 years of age increase lifetime risk from about 7 percent to about 7.3 percent. In contrast to 0.01 percent increases used as guidelines by regulatory agencies concerned with chemical carcinogens, this is a substantial increase.

On the other hand, Xerox mammography practiced in an environment like BCDDP No. 25 is unquestionably superior to palpation and thermography. Thus test accuracy and risk modification are competing considerations to be balanced carefully when considering the use of mammography.[5]

This kind of problem is properly approached using decision analysis techniques applied from the perspective of individual women. In Chapter 9 we used a decision analytic model for the purpose of determining on an annual (or any other periodic) basis the balance of probable benefits against probable costs and radiation risk to asymptomatic women. Through extensive sensitivity analyses in which model parameters, including costs, presumed carcinogenesis rates per rad of exposure, true positive and true negative rates, and possible epidemiological risk levels for women, were systematically varied over their entire ranges of plausible values, we determined conditions under which periodic mammography is appropriate for asymptomatic women. A most important conclusion to be drawn from the analysis is that mammography although an excellent early detection device when true positive and true negative rates are maintained at high levels, should be used sparingly in clinics with low-accuracy rates.

Based on our analysis, annual examinations by clinical palpation and high-quality mammography for most asymptomatic women beginning in the late forties to early fifties are appropriate when true positive and true negative rates for the protocol are, respectively, 82 percent and 98 percent or higher. But the risk-benefit balance for annual screening is not favorable when these rates are substantially lower. When rates for mammography alone fall as low as 60 percent and 50 percent — as have been reported in the literature — mammography should seldom be done because clinical palpation, which is then of comparable accuracy and risk free as well, provides a preferable alternative.

PROTOCOL SELECTION

There are 92 viable detection protocols or strategies using one or more of the three detection modalities: mammography, clinical examination, and thermography. (See Chapter 8.) All 92 protocols were evaluated against one multivariate measure of performance called expected net cost; benefits were incorporated as cost savings. This measure of efficiency accounts for financial costs for detection, biopsy, and treatment; financial benefits in terms of reduced treatment costs with early detection; psychosocial costs for missed cancers and false positive examination; possible radiation risk as an added cost; and frequencies of detected and undetected cancers.[6]

Protocol selection for early detection of breast cancer in asymptomatic women is strongly influenced by a woman's age. It is also strongly influenced by the accuracy with which examination modalities are applied; mammographic accuracy is especially important here, as it is in scheduling examinations. And, of course, the question of who pays what costs is a pivotal one. Accounting for all these factors together, two strategies appear to be optimal or near optimal in most circumstances.

Formal periodic screening is not appropriate for asymptomatic women in their thirties. Incidence rates are extremely low, and mammography is apparently less accurate when breasts are firm and glandular than when they are largely composed of adipose tissue; and palpation is not particularly effective as a free-standing screening modality. (See Chapter 7.) Naturally, women who find lumps in their breast or develop symptoms should be examined upon presentation, but regular screening of asymptomatic women in their thirties is neither optimal nor near optimal. This conclusion holds even when screening is free.

Our conclusions are predictively different for older women. Between the ages of 42 and 48 years or so our analysis shows that the best strategy is biennial examinations using both clinical examination and high-quality mammography. Biopsy would be recommended if either examination were positive.[7] This strategy is appropriate for women of average or higher than average risk.

By the age of 50 years biennial breast examinations with clinical palpation and high-quality mammography for all women are suggested by our benefit-risk analysis. Women in this age range who are at least 50 percent above average risk, or who are especially concerned about undetected cancer, should probably have annual examinations.[8]

In this book we have mapped out a broad set of conditions under which formal periodic screening of asymptomatic women is appropriate. Our conclusions on strategy selection are quite robust. However, they are coupled strongly to the sensitivity and specificity rates for the three tests in one clinical setting. If one were to use instead lower rates for mammography such as those reported elsewhere, detection protocols in which mammography plays a primary role could not be so forcefully recommended.

Thermography, with sensitivity and specificity rates like those obtained at BCDDP No. 25, should play only a minor role as a sensitivity-increasing technique primarily in instances of conflicting findings on the other modalities because the frequency of false positive thermograms is unacceptably high. However, if by technological improvements sensitivity and specificity rates for thermography could be made comparable with those for mammography, it would replace the latter in many protocols for asymptomatic women of all ages because there is no known potential for radiation hazard.

NOTES

1. In this book *true positive rate* and *sensitivity* are used interchangeably as are *true negative rate* and *specificity*. *Sensitivity* refers to the ability of a test modality or a multimodality protocol to detect disease. *Specificity* refers to its ability to select out nondiseased breasts. These two qualities are approximated from statistical data in terms of true positive (*TP*) and true negative (*TN*) rates:

$$TP = \frac{\text{cancer cases screened positive}}{\text{cancer cases}}$$

and

$$TN = \frac{\text{noncancer cases screened negative}}{\text{noncancer cases}}$$

for individual tests or protocols. Other ratios appearing in the literature are the false positive (*FP*) and false negative (*FN*) rates. These are related to the first two as follows: $FP = 1 - TN$ and $FN = 1 - TP$.

2. The Division of Health Care Research, Preventive Medicine, Washington University, has under way a survey of radiological centers. Results to date show clearly that centers typically do not have the data necessary to calculate their true positive and true negative rates. Neither do they engage in patient follow-up and case review to the extent necessary to generate such data. Hopefully, such practices will eventually be implemented. In their absence our findings on which features to look for to optimize detection practices are especially important.

3. Incidence rates among asymptomatic women are very low. At BCDDP No. 25 between 20 and 25 new cancers were detected annually among approximately 10,000 women for an incidence rate of about 0.25 percent. In ordinary radiological practices between 100 and 600 breast examinations are done annually [Jans and Ohlhaber 1979]. And a large fraction of these are for symptomatic women. Thus most centers will probably recommend biopsy for only 5 or 10 asymptomatic women in a year. If all of these were not followed, a great deal of information would be lost.

A large fraction of symptomatic women X-rayed will undergo breast biopsy. Quality of service would likely be enhanced if a fraction of these cases were followed through pathology as well.

4. Low-dose mammography can reduce exposure levels to less than half a rad per breast. Radiation risk is presumably proportionally reduced under these circumstances but is not eliminated. On the other hand, the value of mammography lies primarily in the quality of the image and its interpretation. We found no data directly comparing sensitivity and specificity rates for the two mammographic techniques.

5. We cannot emphasize too strongly the critical role of accuracy in mammography. No matter how one varies the other model parameters, accuracy is a central consideration. Inaccuracy results in missed early cancers and more negative biopsies with all the financial and psychosocial costs they entail. Compared with accuracy, the question of whether to use Xerox mammography, at about 1 rad of exposure per breast per examination, or low-dose film/screen mammography, with less than half the dosage, appears to be a minor consideration.

6. Psychosocial costs cannot be estimated with precision. In Appendix B we document the process by which such costs can be approximated in terms of what economists call opportunity costs or shadow prices, and we provide ranges of estimates for the costs used in our work; the estimates are extracted from the liability and economics literature. Because precision is impossible, we treat such costs as parameters of analysis and investigate the implications of inaccuracy on choices. Our recommendations are based on having found broad ranges of stability in these relationships.

7. The definitions of *positive* and *negative examinations* were given previously. See Table 7.4.

8. Because no variables other than age were found in BCDDP No. 25 data to contribute to increased risk, we have no original statistical basis for presuming elevated risk for any age group. We can only suggest that there may be factors that would contribute to elevated age-specific risk. If risk elevation of 50 percent could be documented for a woman, annual screening would be in order.

REFERENCES

Berlin NI (1978) Breast cancer screening: the facts in perspective. Oncology News, 28 February, 1978, p. 2.

Boice, JD, Land CE, Shore RE, Norman JE, and Tokunaga M (1979) Risk of breast cancer following low-dose radiation. Diagnostic Radiology 131:589-597.

Culliton B (1977) Mammography controversy: NIH's entree into evaluating technology. Science 198: 171-173.

Egan RL, Mosteller RC, Stephens CD, Egan KL (1977) Risk, biopsy, and breast cancer: new approach through combined epidemiologic, clinical, and X-ray indications. Breast: Diseases of the Breast 4(1) n.p.

Fox H, Moskowitz M, Saenger E, Kerelakes J, Milbrath J, and Goodman M (1978) Benefit/risk analysis of aggressive mammographic screening. Radiology 128:359-365.

Gohagan JK, Rodes ND, Blackwell CW, Darby WP, Farrell C, Herder TJ, Pearson DK, Spitznagel EL, Wallace D (1980) Individual and combined effectiveness of palpation, thermography, and mammography in breast cancer screening. Preventive Medicine 9:713-721.

Gohagan JK, Spitznagel EL, Darby WP, Feiner J (1981) Optimal strategies for breast cancer detection. Proceedings International Conference on Systems Science in Health Care. New York, Pergamon Press.

Gold R (1977) Enlightenment at last! Mammographic depth dose versus surface exposure. Medical Imaging, 4th Quarter, n.p.

Hicks MJ, Davis JR, Layton JM, Present AJ (1979) Sensitivity of mammography and physical examination of the breast for detecting breast cancer. JAMA 242:2080-2083.

Jans RG, Ohlhaber TR (1979) Reduced dose mammography . . . results of a nationwide study, *in* Logan WW and Muntz EP (eds), Reduced dose mammography. New York, Masson.

Menitoff R (1978) A decision analytic approach to the evaluation of alternative breast cancer screening practices and strategies. Masters thesis. Sever Institute of Technology School of Engineering and Applied Science, Washington University, St. Louis, Mo.

United Nations Scientific Committee on the Effects of Atomic Radiation (UNSCEAR) (1977) Sources and Effects of Ionizing Radiation. New York, United Nations.

Upton AC, Beebe GW, Brown JM, et al. (1977) Report of NCI Ad Hoc Working Group on the risks associated with mammography in screening for the detection of breast cancer. J Natl Canc Inst 59:481-493.

11

Early Diagnosis and Therapeutic Alternatives

Harvey R. Butcher
Walter F. Ballinger
Marc K. Wallack

Breast cancer has been described throughout recorded history, but data regarding its epidemiological characteristics have been accumulated only in recent times. Much is now known about the natural occurrence of the disease, its untreated behavior, and its relative incidence in different parts of the world. Its etiology remains obscure, but a vast body of evidence has been accumulated regrading its association with viral particles in the experimental animal, in human breast milk, and in some human breast cancers. Furthermore, its association with the female hormonal milieu is apparent, and the relationship between the presence or absence of estrogen and progesterone receptors and the characteristics of breast cancer has been an important advance in determining prognosis in both individuals and large populations of patients.

More than 90,000 new cases of breast cancer occur every year in the United States, making this the most common cancer in women in this country. There are 35,000 deaths due to this disease per year, making it the most deadly cancer in women. Stated another way, approximately 25 percent of women who die of cancer, die of breast cancer. Finally, approximately 1 in 15 women in this country will develop breast cancer.

DISEASE STAGING

It has been helpful to clinicians and investigators to develop a reliable method of staging the disease at the time of first appearance of the patient in the physician's office or at various intervals in the course of treatment. Such information permits valuable references when related to the historical data already available regarding untreated disease. Because one cannot study the course of the disease in a control population of untreated women, such information is based upon past data. This probably introduces a biased interpretation of treatment results since it can be inferred that the natural course of the disease might have changed over decades.

Although a number of staging schemata have been developed, it is appropriate here to describe that proposed first by the International Union against Cancer in 1954 and adopted by the American Joint Committee for Cancer Staging and Results in 1962. Since that time many changes have occurred, but the basic format remains. The system is based, first, on the stage of the primary tumor itself; second, on the presence or absence of regional nodal metastasis; and, finally, on the presence or absence of distal metastasis to such organs as bone, lung, and liver. Utilizing this TNM system (T[tumor], N[node], M[metastasis]), it is possible to characterize four stages of the disease. Thus, T1 N0 M0 would represent minimal cancer with no nodal or distant spread. In contrast, $T_3 N_2 M_1$ indicates that a large tumor is present in the breast with significant nodal metastasis as well as the presence of distal metastasis—that is, advanced breast cancer. Other clinical diagnostic criteria that have been used for many years were modified by Haagensen and Stout in the 1940s and led to certain standards of inoperability for significant control of disease. These included such signs as extensive edema of the skin over the breast, satellite nodules in the skin, reddening of the skin of the breast (inflammatory carcinoma), and supraclavicular nodes palpable clinically.

The size of the tumor is of prognostic significance; in general, tumors less than 2 cm in size have a prognosis significantly better than those larger. Nevertheless, it is now well recognized that there may well be separate subpopulations including small (aggressive) tumors that metastasize early and large tumors that metastasize late. Thus, clinical staging simply provides a time-zero reference at the initial diagnosis of breast cancer and a baseline from which the choice and the effect of oncologic therapy may be determined.

Following the biopsy, with or without acquisition of material from the axilla, the pathologist is able to provide more accurate information regarding staging and prognosis of the disease. For example, patients with four or more positive axillary nodes have a significantly poorer prognosis than those with fewer than four nodes involved. Quite obviously, those with clinically and histologically negative axillary lymph nodes have a better prognosis than even those with one positive node. Thus, staging using ±4 nodes is useful in developing patient populations for purposes both of study and therapy.

Another method of staging has resulted from the increasingly widespread appreciation of tumor biology and the behavior of individual cell populations within tumors. Although at one time there appeared to be some enthusiasm for recognizing a supposed protective affect of a high lymphocyte population in and around tumors, this does not appear to be statistically valid today. As information accumulates regarding doubling time of tumors, certain histologic characteristics as well as the presence or absence of hormone receptor sites on the cells will provide increasing support for the theory of variable aggressiveness of individual tumor populations. Furthermore, such knowledge will undoubtedly have a significant effect upon the planning of therapeutic programs for individual patients.

THERAPEUTIC ALTERNATIVES

At the present time the therapeutic primary alternatives in the management of women with breast cancer apparently confined to the breast and possibly the axilla include the following:

1. Radical mastectomy,
2. Total mastectomy and axillary dissection,
3. Segmental mastectomy with axillary dissection, and
4. Tylectomy (removal of the mass only) and radiation therapy.

Postoperative radiation, chemotherapy, and hormonal therapy are adjuvant therapies.

SURGERY

Radical mastectomy removes the entire breast and overlying skin, the pectoralis major and minor muscles, and the axillary contents in continuity. Reported by Halsted [1894] and Meyer [1894], radical mastectomy became the traditional form of therapy for all women with breast cancer in the first 50 years of the twentieth century because of apparently less frequent chest wall recurrence. The apparent improvement in survival that was noted during this time was, however, related for the most part to earlier diagnosis and more careful selection of cases for operation. Haagensen and Stout [1943], for example, in establishing the Columbia system of staging, defined those women with breast cancer most likely to have long-term survival after radical operation. By limiting radical mastectomy to this group of women, results appeared improved. Only in the past 20 years has radical mastectomy been subjected to unbiased testing by proper staging and randomized trials.

Total mastectomy with axillary dissection (modified radical mastectomy) has become more and more popular among surgeons in recent years. It differs from the classical radical mastectomy in that the pectoralis major muscle is not removed. The Patey operation removes the pectoralis minor muscle, while the Auchincloss version simply retracts the latter muscle in performing the axillary dissection. The end results of either procedure are similar to those following the classic radical mastectomy. The advantages of the modified radical mastectomy include less likelihood of significant swelling of the arm, stronger shoulder function, and a better cosmetic result. There is a theoretical disadvantage in that the high nodes (those proximal to the medial border of the pectoralis minor) are not removed, particularly with the Auchincloss version of the operation, but no investigator has yet shown that this in any way alters the end results. This procedure is the preferred operation of most surgeons today [Special Report 1979].

Total mastectomy without axillary dissection is called simple mastectomy. Although few surgeons believe that simple mastectomy is superior to more radical operations, evidence has begun to accrue in support of its efficacy in treating clinical Stage I cancer of the breast. A randomized trial initiated by the National Surgical Adjuvant Breast Project in 1971 compared radical mastectomy, total mastectomy, and total mastectomy with radiation in the treatment of clinical Stage I mammary cancer [Fisher et al. 1977a]. Those patients treated by total mastectomy alone who in follow-up developed biopsy-proven axillary metastases had axillary dissection. The end results to date have been the same in the three treatment groups. However, total mastectomy alone cannot be recommended at present because of the importance of pathologic staging of the axillary nodes. The improved disease-free interval among patients with axillary nodal metastases treated by adjuvant chemotherapy makes at least partial axillary dissection mandatory [Bonnadonna et al. 1976, Fisher et al. 1975].

To investigate the potential of reducing the severity of surgery for women with limited disease and the potential for a satisfactory cosmetic result, the National Surgical Adjuvant Breast Project has under way a randomized trial comparing total mastectomy with axillary dissection, segmental mastectomy (removal of a breast segment only) with axillary dissection, and a segmental mastectomy with axillary dissection followed by mammary radiation. Meaningful end results are not yet available. Segmental mastectomy with axillary dissection cannot yet be recommended except to patients willing to enter the protocol.

IMMUNOLOGY AND TUMOR MARKERS

Moore and Foote [1949] discussed the relatively favorable prognosis of medullary carcinoma of the breast because of lymphocytic infiltrates present around the tumor. Later, Black et al. [1953] described a more favorable prognosis associated with a regional lymph node pattern of sinus histocytosis. More recent studies of the histology of the regional lymph node in breast cancer have not agreed as to the clinical significance of various lymphocytic patterns. For example, Tsakraklides et al. [1976]

studied 303 cases and found no prognostic value in assessment of regional lymph node histology. Thus, the issue remains to be resolved.

In the search for tumor markers in breast cancer, a variety of approaches have been used including analysis of metabolic by-products, oncofetal antigens, virus particles, plasma proteins, hormones, and cell-associated components of breast cancer tissue. The markers that are the most frequently encountered in disseminated breast cancer were human chorionic gonadotropin (HCG) and carcinoembryonic antigen (CEA). These tumor markers were elevated in 47 percent and 65 percent of advanced cancer patients, respectively [Tormey et al. 1977].

CEA is a glycoprotein that has been detected in a variety of malignant and nonmalignant disease states. With respect to breast cancer, CEA is not detectable in all cases but when present can be a valuable tool for monitoring the patient. Steward et al. [1974] found CEA titers to parallel patient response to treatment with increasing values during therapy showing a poor response and low titers in patients with good responses. Moreover, in a large study of 824 postoperative patients, Myers et al. [1977] found 60.2 percent of patients with Stage IV breast cancer to have elevated CEAs with CEA levels correlating with disease recurrence and progression. Thus, CEA can be used to both mark response to therapy and assess recurrence.

The presence of elevated levels of HCG in any condition other than pregnancy is considered abnormal. The recent development by Braunstein et al. [1973] of a sensitive radioimmunoassay has revealed that HCG may be elevated in serum of patients with types of cancer other than trophoblastic neoplasms. By this procedure any value above 5 mIU/ml of serum is considered elevated. Initial studies indicated that greater than 40 percent of patients with metastatic breast cancer had serum levels above 5 mIU/ml [Tormey et al. 1975, Tormey and Waalkes 1976]. Further clinical investigations have since shown that patients with metastatic breast cancer who had elevated pretreatment levels of HCG and have either responded or progressed with therapy had corresponding appropriately measurable changes in HCG values. This suggests that HCG may also be of potential value as a biomarker under these circumstances.

The probability of one biomarker fulfilling all requirements to serve as an adjunctive test for staging and monitoring the breast cancer throughout its course appears unlikely. As a result both hCG and CEA should be used as potential markers in all patients with breast cancer in anticipation that a group of tests will provide a broader coverage as compared with using one alone.

Both HCG and CEA can provide data regarding the progression of breast cancer with increases in these markers signifying progression of disease. Commonly used assays to provide overall data regarding immunologic competence include delayed hypersensitivity, skin tests with common-recall antigens, lymphocyte counts, concentrations of T and B cells, in vitro lymphocyte transformation assays with mitogens and common-recall antigens, and serum immunoglobulin levels. Failure to demonstrate normal patterns by the above methods may indicate compromise of immunologic potential, although this area is still quite controversial.

Significant impairment of skin test reactivity to a battery of common antigens was observed in metastatic breast cancer by Nemoto et al. [1974]. Use of skin testing as a prognostic indicator, however, has generally met with unfavorable results because many patients with recurrent disease may show normal reactivity [Stein et al. 1976].

Quantitation of T- and B-lymphocytes in breast cancer has produced somewhat disappointing results. A number of studies have failed to detect any direct correlation between percentage of T cells and clinical status [Wanebo et al. 1976].

Circulating immunoglobulins have also been measured in breast cancer. Meyer et al. [1973], in an uncontrolled study, noted increased IgA in radiation-treated, disease-free patients, with disease recurrence correlated with decreased IgA levels.

A critical problem in evaluating any immunologic data in cancer patients is posed by the destructive affects of radiation or chemotherapy on the immune system. Stjensward et al. [1972] examined patients with mammary carcinoma before and after radiation and noted lymphopenia, depressed delayed hypersensitivity responses, and shifts in T and B cell concentrations lasting at least one year after treatment.

Basic laboratory immunologic assays have been applied to human breast cancer in the hope of further defining an immunologic aspect to the disease and also providing clinically relevant data. The specificity of the immunologic responses observed in these studies has not been determined, and the clinical significance of the data has received little attention. The presence of antitumor antibody has been examined by immunofluorescence and complement fixation studies [Humphrey et al. 1974, Priori et al. 1971]. Although antibody has been noted, the specificity and clinical relevance are not clarified.

Cell-mediated immunity has been examined by in vivo and in vitro methods. Stewart and Orizaga [1971] skin tested 56 patients with extracts of their own tumor and suggested that the lack of delayed hypersensitivity reactions observed in 12 patients correlated with the presence of anaplastic tumor, regional node metastasis, and poor survival.

In vitro methods of evaluating cellular immunity to breast cancer included assays for lymphocyte tumor-directed cytotoxicity, lymphocyte transformation stimulated by tumor cells, and inhibition or rucocyte migration. At present the significance of such findings is not clear.

Immunotherapy, a relatively new addition to the treatment of cancer, may be generally classified as passive or active, specific or nonspecific. Passive immunotherapy refers to approaches in which the patient is given immunologic agents such as whole lymphoid cells, sera, or lymphoid cell products that are thought to have antitumor capability. In active specific immunotherapy the host is stimulated by an administration of tumor antigens to mount an immune response that specifically causes tumor cell death. The nonspecific immunotherapy used in most clinical trials consists of administration of agents such as *Bacillus* Calmette-Guerin (BCG); *Corynebacterium parvum* (*C. parvum*); and methanol-extractable residue of BCG called MER, or Lavamisole, a synthetic antihelmintic drug. Very few of the studies using these techniques in the treatment of breast cancer have been randomized, and, therefore, results are difficult to interpret. At best one could say the approach appears promising from a theoretical perspective, but its efficacy in breast cancer needs to be determined in well-designed randomized prospective trials.

HORMONE RECEPTORS

Although endocrine therapy for advanced breast cancer is not new, our understanding of how hormones effect the growth of breast tumor cells and the application of these principles to treatment strategies have changed over the past several years. The use of estrogen receptors (ERs) to select endocrine-responsive tumors is routine in all breast cancer patients. The ER assay may be performed on as little as 100 to 200 mg fresh or frozen tissue. The tissue cytosol is obtained by homogenization of the tumor tissue, followed by incubation with tritium-labeled estradiol. Labeled unbound hormone is then removed from the incubation mixture by absorption to dextran coated charcoal [King 1975]. Cytoplasmic levels of ER protein in a particular specimen may be measured and are usually reported as femtomoles of estradiol bound per mg of total protein. A tumor with a level of less than 3 femtomoles is usually considered ER negative, but definition of positive and negative may vary from lab to lab [Wittliff and Savlov 1978].

Collective data from over 400 treatment trials from 14 institutions using different ER assay methods shows that tumor ER status correlates well with response to hormone therapy [McGuire et al. 1975]. These data show that patients having tumors that contain ER have a 55 to 60 percent response rate to additive endocrine therapy. A more striking relationship is observed for ER negative tumors in that less than 10 percent of these patients have objective remissions with endocrine therapy. It is clear, therefore, that the ER assay is most helpful when the tumor is receptor negative [Walt et al. 1976]. Clinicians can exclude with considerable confidence those patients with negative assays from endocrine therapy.

In order to improve on the ER assay applicability, studies have been done to show that tumors with more ER-positive cells and a higher absolute ER level might be more responsive to endocrine therapy, although preliminary observation does not reveal a correlation between the level of ER and response to therapy [McGuire et al. 1975]. McGuire, in a recent analysis of 111 patients with receptor assay on biopsy of metastases have shown that the higher the ER level, the better the response to endocrine therapy. Patients with levels greater than 100 femtomoles per mg of protein had an 81 percent response rate to endocrine manipulation.

In normal target tissue such as the uterus, one can only obtain a biologic effect from progesterone by priming the tissue with estrogen. This is explained by the fact that estrogen induces the synthesis of progesterone receptors (PgRs). Since PgRs are an end product of estrogen action, the measurement of PgRs in breast tissue specimens has been proposed as a method of determining the presence of an intact estrogen response pathway, thereby providing a better marker of the hormone dependence of the tumor. Several laboratories have been measuring ERs and PgRs in breast tumors and correlating the results with response to hormone therapy. These laboratories have shown that about one third of tumors have neither receptor, one third have only ER, and one third have both receptors. These data show an increased remission rate (as high as 79 percent) in tumors containing both receptors [Young et al. 1978]. Thus, quantitating the absolute levels of ERs and measuring the PgRs enhances the clinicians' ability to select patients for endocrine therapy. It is not clear, however, if measurement of PgRs provides additional information beyond that given by the correlation between absolute ER level and tumor response. Since tumors with high levels of ER are more likely to contain PgR, these assays may actually be identifying the same groups of patients [Osborne and McGuire 1978].

Other than predicting tumor response in patients with advanced metastatic breast cancer, analysis of the ER data in patients undergoing curative surgery for primary breast cancer has led to another important use for the ER assay [Knight et al. 1978]. In 190 patients of surgically treated breast cancer, patients with ER-negative tumors had recurrences at a significantly faster rate than those with ER-positive tumors. In this series 36 percent of all patients with ER-negative tumors had recurrent disease compared with only 17 percent in the ER-positive group [Knight et al. 1977]. Thus, the ER status of a primary breast tumor is a prognostic marker for rate of recurrence independent of other variables.

These observations are of tremendous clinical importance. First, because of the prognostic importance of ERs, all future adjuvant treatment studies of primary breast cancer should include ER status. Second, the ER status of a primary tumor may help in the design of new adjuvant therapy strategies by delineating patients who are at high risk for recurrence.

EARLY DETECTION

The hope has always been present among clinicians that earlier diagnosis will lead to a higher rate of "curability" and reduced overall mortality for breast cancer. Thus, the clinical goal is to identify those tumors with limited potential for metastasis in the earlier stages to achieve a near 100 percent "cure" rate. (Of course, tumors that can be identified as highly aggressive and that metastasize earlier would need to be studied further for the best possible form of adjuvant therapy since they undoubtedly are systemic and have spread far from their site of origin by the time they are first discovered.)

Thus, increasing attention has been given in recent years to methods of early detection of breast cancer. Although there are a number of statistical biases that exist in most screening and early detection clinics, it would appear that it is not only possible to diagnose tumors earlier but, at least in some groups of patients, to reduce mortality due to tumor by early detection and proper treatment. As a result of early studies, chiefly that of the NY Health Insurance Plan in 1963, a number of model breast cancer detection centers (Breast Cancer Detection Demonstration Projects [BCDDPs]) were established by the National Cancer Institute and the American Cancer Society. Although all final opinions are not in, it would appear that these clinics have demonstrated that the triad of adequate, periodic and systematic self-examination, annual clinical examination by a highly trained health care professional, and mammography when indicated will yield a significant number of breast cancers that might otherwise have remained undetected for much longer periods of time—and might have metastasized in that time.

Thus, as more is learned of the characteristics of breast disease in large populations (epidemiology) and in individual cell populations (tumor biology), as well as in early detection of mammary cancer, treatment modalities utilizing surgical and nonsurgical means should become even more successful in control of the disease.

REFERENCES

Black MM, Kerpe S, Speer FD (1953) Lymph node structure in patients with cancer of the breast. Amer J Path 29:505.

Bonnadonna G, et al. (1976) Combination chemotherapy as an adjuvant treatment in operable breast cancer. New Engl J Med 294:405-410.

Braunstein GD, Vaitukaitis JL, Carbone PP, et al. (1973) Ectopic production of human chorionic gonadotrophin by neoplasms. Ann Intern Med 78:39-45.

Fisher B, Montague E, Redmond C, et al. (1977a) Comparison of radical mastectomy with alternative treatments for primary breast cancer. Cancer 39:2827-2839.

Fisher B, et al. (1977b) L-Pam in the management of primary breast cancer. Cancer 39:2882–2903.

Fisher B, et al. (1975) L-phenylalanine mustard (L-Pam) in the management of primary breast cancer. New Engl J Med 292:117-122.

Fisher ER, Gregorio R, Redmond C, et al. (1976) Pathologic findings from the Natonal Surgical Adjuvant Breast Cancer Project (Protocol #4). The significance of regional lymph node histology other than sinus histiocytosis in invasive mammary cancer. Am J Clin Pathol 65:21-30.

Haagensen CD, Stout AP (1943) Carcinoma of the breast; criteria of operability. Ann Surg 118:859-870.

Halsted WS (1894) The results of operations for cure of cancer of the breast performed at the Johns Hopkins Hospital from June 1889 to January 1894. Johns Hopkins Hospital Rep 4:297-350.

Humphrey LJ, Estes NC, Morse PA, Jr, Jewell WR, Boudet RA, Hudson MJK (1974) Serum antibody in patients with mammary disease. Cancer 34:1516-1520.

King RJB (1975) Clinical relevance of steroid-receptor measurements in tumors. Cancer Treat Rev 2:273-293.

Knight WA, III, Livingston RB, Gregory EJ, et al. (1978) Absent estrogen receptor and decreased survival in human breast cancer. Proceedings from the 14th Annual Meeting of the American Society of Clinical Oncology, C342. Washington, D.C., American Society of Clinical Oncology.

Knight WA, III, Livingston RB, Gregory EJ, et al. (1977) Estrogen receptors as an independent prognostic factor for early recurrence in breast cancer. Cancer 37:4669.

McGuire WL, Carbone PP, Vollmer EP (1975) Estrogen receptors in human breast cancer. New York, Raven Press.

McGuire, WL, Horwitz KB, Zava DT, Garola RE, Chamness GC (1978) Hormones in breast cancer: update 1978. Metabolism 27:487-501.

Meyer KK, Mackler GL, Beck WC (1973) Increased IgA in women free of recurrence after mastectomy and radiation. Arch Surg 107:159-161.

Meyer W (1894) An improved method of radical operation for carcinoma of the breast. NY Med Rec 46:746-755.

Moore OS, Foote FW, Jr. (1949) The relatively favorable prognosis of medullary carcinoma of the breast. Cancer 2:635-642.

Myers RE, Sutherland DJA, Malkin A, et al. (1977) CEA in breast cancer. International Conference on Clinical Uses of Carcinoembryonic Antigens. Cancer 42:1520-1526.

Nemoto T, Han T, Minowada J, Angkor U, Chamberlain WA, Dav TL, August W (1974) Cell-mediated immune status of breast cancer patients: evaluation by skin tests, lymphocyte stimulation and counts of rosette-forming cells. J Natl Cancer Inst 53:641-645.

Osborne CK, McGuire WL (1978) Current use of steroid hormonal receptor assays in the treatment of breast cancer. Surgical Clinics of North America 58:777-788.

Priori ES, Seaman G, Smockowski HS, et al. (1971) Immunofluorescence studies of sera of patients with breast cancer. Cancer 29: 1462-1471.

Special Report — Treatment of Primary Breast Cancer (1979) New Engl J Med 301: 340.

Stein JA, Adler A, Ben Efraim SB, Maor M (1976) Immunocompetence, immunosuppression, and human breast cancer. I. An analysis of their relationship by known parameters of cell-mediated immunity in well-defined clinical stages of disease. Cancer 38:1171-1187.

Steward AM, Nixon D, Zamcheck AA (1974) Carcinoembryonic antigen in breast cancer patients: serum levels and disease progress. Cancer 33:1246-1252.

Stewart THM, Orizaga M (1971) The presence of delayed hypersensitivity reactions in patients toward cellular extracts of their malignant tumors. Cancer 28:1472-1478.

Stjensward J, Jondal M, Vanky F, Wigzell H, Sealy R (1972) Lymphopenia and change in distribution of human B- and T-lymphocytes in peripheral blood induced by irradiation for mammary carcinoma. Lancet 1:1342-1356.

Tormey DC, Waalkes TP (1976) Biochemical markers in cancer of the breast. Recent Results Cancer Res 57:78-94.

Tormey DC, Waalkes TP, Ahmann D, et al. (1975) Biological markers in breast carcinoma. I. Incidence of abnormalities of CEA, HCG, three polyamines and three minor nucleosides. Cancer 35:1095-1100.

Tormey DC, Waalkes TP, Snyder JJ, et al. (1977) Biological markers in breast carcinoma. III. Clinical correlations with carcinoembryonic antigen. Cancer 39:2397-2404.

Tsakraklides V, Olson P, Kersey JH, Good RA (1974) Prognostic significance of the regional lymph node histology in cancer of the breast. Cancer 34:1259-1267.

Walt AJ, Singhakowinta A, Brooks SC, et al. (1976) The surgical implications of estrophile protein estimations in carcinoma of the breast. Surgery 80:506-512.

Wanebo HJ, Thaler T, Urban J, Oettgen H (1976) Immunobiology of operable breast cancer: an assessment of biologic risk by immunoparameters. Ann Surg 184(3):258-267.

Wise L, Mason VY, Ackerman LV (1971) Local excision and irradiation: an alternative method for the treatment of early mammary cancer. Ann Surg 174:392-401.

Wittliff JL, Savlov ED (1978) Biochemical basis for the selection of hormonal manipulation in the patient with breast carcinoma. Int J Radiat Oncol Biol Phys 4:463-467.

Young PCM, Einhorn LH, Ehrlich CE, et al. (1978) Progesterone receptors (PgR) as a marker of hormone-responsive breast cancer. Proc Am Assoc Can Res 19:204.

Appendix A: Screening Forms

FINAL OBJECTIVES AND GUIDELINES FOR THE NATIONAL BREAST CANCER DETECTION DEMONSTRATION PROJECT (NBCDDP)

Operational

1. Recruit 10,000 asymptomatic, nonpregnant women between the ages of 35 and 74 years in each of the 27 projects over a two-year period for a total of 270,000 women in the program.
2. Screen each of these women with history, physical examination, mammography, and thermography, each independently obtained and interpreted in accordance with guidelines for specific age groups.
3. Refer these screenees for either surgical consultation, (that is, biopsy or aspiration), early recall, or annual rescreen on the basis of overall evaluation of the combined screening modalities.
4. Assist all screenees in entering the medical care system.
5. Inform all screenees and their physicians of the results of each examination.
6. Examine all screenees annually by all three modalities according to age group guidelines for a total of five annual examinations.
7. Follow each screenee annually for five years after the five annual screenings.
8. Provide information as to the usefulness of ACS volunteers in recruiting, recalling, and follow-up of all the participating women.
9. Utilize the lowest practicable level of radiation exposure consistent with good (mammographic) image quality.
10. Prepare a complete set of data forms on each screenee. Data sets will be sent to a data management center for processing and management.

Educational

1. Improve the quality of mammography, physical examination, thermography, and histopathologic diagnosis.
2. Maintain a quality control program for the pathological interpretation of benign and malignant breast lesions identified in these projects.

This material was taken from the U.S. DHEW/PHS/NIH 1978 Manual of Procedures and Operations for the National Cancer Institute and the American Cancer Society Breast Cancer Detection Demonstration Project.

3. Maintain a quality control program for imagery and for radiation monitoring practices.
4. Teach women breast self-examination and encourage them to perform it regularly.
5. Explore the advisability of using nonphysician personnel in screening examinations (that is, doing a physical examination, taking an X ray).

Scientific and Evaluative

1. Identify the demographic characteristics of the screenees and other factors such as reasons for entry to study, continuation of self-examination, etcetera.
2. Identify etiologic factors associated with breast cancer and with benign breast disease through a retrospective epidemiological case-control study utilizing breast cancer cases from this program.
3. Identify the size, nodal involvement, and pathology of breast cancer especially with respect to detection modality.
4. Tabulate the results of screening modalities as applied in this program.
5. Develop and evaluate technology for monitoring radiation exposures through use of ionization chambers and thermoluminescent dosimetry.

If the participant does not read or understand English, an interpreter should fully explain the information on this form.

Although you have signed consent forms at the time of your previous examinations, you should read this form carefully and then decide whether you will give your informed consent to continue your participation in the Breast Cancer Detection Demonstration Project. As you are aware, this screening program has been modified periodically. These changes reflect the continuing assessment of information concerning risks and benefits.

Women who participate in the program can receive up to four types of examinations, in five annual screenings. The examinations will be conducted by physicians or specially trained nurses and technicians under the supervision of a physician. You are encouraged to ask questions concerning any examinations you will be given.

Some participants will also be asked to answer a follow-up letter or telephone call once a year for an additional period of time to determine the effectiveness of the screening program.

PART I—RISKS AND BENEFITS OF BREAST CANCER SCREENING

Nearly one out of thirteen American women will develop breast cancer at some time during their lifetime. Breast Cancer is the primary cause of death from cancer in women of all ages and is the leading cause of all deaths among women 40-44 years old. During 1978, 34,000 women are estimated to die of breast cancer in the United States. Early diagnosis is believed to be important because there is greater potential for effective treatment.

A controlled study started in 1963 showed that a screening procedure that used a combination of mammography and physical examination resulted in a decreased mortality (death rate) from breast cancer for women age 50 and older. Neither this study nor any other data to date show a similar decrease in mortality for women below the age of 50. Mammography has improved technically since the controlled screening study was conducted, and might now result in increased benefits to all women, including those under 50 years of age. However, such an improvement in benefits has not yet been proven for younger women.

The risks and benefits of the four types of examinations are:

1. Clinical History. (A medical questionnaire about you and your family.) There are no risks in collecting medical information about participants. The benefits can be great, for past medical history can provide good information for diagnostic purposes or for estimating risks.

2. Physical Examination of the Breast. (Observation and palpation [touching] of the breast.) Regular, careful physical examinations can lead to the discovery of breast cancers. Undergoing this examination is not harmful.

178

3. Thermography. (A photograph to identify differences in skin temperature of the breast.) This examination does not produce any risk of cancer or other known harmful results. The contribution of thermography as it is used in breast cancer screening has not been proven scientifically. This procedure for routine screening will be phased out in the near future.

4. Mammography. (X-rays of the breast.) Mammography is a medical technique which uses X-rays to find and diagnose conditions that are not normal in the breasts. X-rays are ionizing radiation and studies have shown exposure to such radiation in large doses can cause breast cancer many years after original exposure. The mammographic examination in the BCDDP requires two X-ray exposures of each breast with the average delivered dose per two-view examination calculated to be approximately one rad or less (average dose absorbed at mid breast for a 6 cm. breast). The radiation dose which you as an individual woman will receive cannot be specified precisely; however, the radiation dosage from the mammographic examination given in these BCDDPs is monitored yearly in detail at each project by specially qualified personnel, with spot checks at all projects twice a month to document consistency of the doses being delivered. The output exposure of the machine which will be used for your examination was determined to approximate a mid breast absorbed dose of _____ rads per two-view examination. You are free to ask questions concerning the X-ray dose you receive from your mammographic examinations.

Although the risk of a single mammographic examination at a dose of one rad or less to an individual woman is very small, exposure does accumulate with each additional examination. With the small doses of radiation to the breast involved in mammography, the hypothetical risks are generally thought to be acceptably small in relation to the expected benefits of the procedure for the detection of cancer in women of your age group.

PART II—ELIGIBILITY CRITERIA FOR SCREENING

Because of questions raised about mammography and breast cancer screening, a special panel composed of scientists, epidemiologists, physicians, and representatives of the clergy, the legal profession, and the lay public, examined the issues in September 1977. Based on the findings of this panel, the following criteria were established for the BCDDP.

- It should be understood that when there are any signs or symptoms of breast cancer, mammography is an accepted part of the complete diagnostic procedure and should not be confused with a routine screening examination. Thermography, likewise, may be used for diagnostic purposes.

- For routine screening purposes, mammography may be used only as follows:

    1. Women 50 years of age (current age) or older may be given mammographic examinations as a part of the routine screening process, in conjunction with the physical examination.

    2. For all women 40 through 49 years of age (current age), routine annual screening by mammography will be discontinued except where there exists:

        a. A personal history of breast cancer, or

        b. A history of breast cancer in the screenee's immediate family (mother/sisters).

    3. Women 35-39 years of age may be given mammography in this Project only if they have a personal history of breast cancer. All other routine mammography screening in this age group will be discontinued.

    4. For women under 50 years of age who did not meet the above criteria, the government will not support the cost of any mammogram provided at the individual screenee's request when there are no abnormal breast findings. Written requests from the screenee's personal physician for her to have a mammogram will be honored by the project.

In each of the above instances, appropriate informed consent must be obtained.

PART III—GENERAL INFORMATION

• You are encouraged to continue in the screening program for clinical history and physical examination and to participate in the follow-up interviews even if thermography or mammography are not included in your examination. You are also encouraged to perform regularly the breast self-examination which you were taught in this program and to discuss with a physician any changes which you might observe.

• The use of modern mammography might find very small breast abnormalities which can be difficult to diagnose on pathological examination. If you are referred to your physician with a recommendation for biopsy, you may wish to discuss with your physician the desirability of additional pathology consultation on the biopsy before undergoing further surgical treatment. Physicians can differ in their interpretation of such small abnormalities.

DEPARTMENT OF HEALTH, EDUCATION, AND WELFARE	1. OFFICE (01-02)		FORM APPROVED O.M.B. NO. 68-R1377
PUBLIC HEALTH SERVICE			
NATIONAL INSTITUTES OF HEALTH	2. ACCESSION NUMBER (03-08)		
NATIONAL CANCER INSTITUTE – AMERICAN CANCER SOCIETY			
BREAST CANCER DETECTION DEMONSTRATION PROJECT			ANNUAL VISIT SERIES NUMBER
INFORMED CONSENT RECORD	3. FORM TYPE (09-10)	9 1	4. EXAM NUMBER (11-12)

PART IV – INFORMATION GATHERED DURING SCREENING PROGRAM

Women participating in the program will be informed of the results of the screening tests and of any additional tests they agree to take. The screenees' physicians will be notified when biopsy or aspiration is recommended and the women will be referred to their private physicians for further consultation and examination. Any personal information obtained about participants will be kept confidential, but such information can be used for statistical reports and for other scientific purposes concerned with breast cancer. Under federal regulations participants are protected from voluntary disclosure of this information for purposes other than scientific or research.

PART V – CONSENT SECTION

I have read and understand the statements on the four pages of this form, and I agree to participate in the National Cancer Institute-American Cancer Society breast cancer screening program to detect breast cancer at an early stage.

I give my permission to those locally in charge of the screening program to exchange information and materials regarding my case with my private physician or the clinic or hospital to which I may be referred.

Each of the procedures has been explained to me, along with the accompanying risks and benefits. I have been offered the opportunity to make inquiries to my personal physician or members of the program staff concerning those examinations, and they have been answered to my satisfaction. I understand that I may ask additional questions about the program at any time.

I understand that this consent form pertains only to this breast cancer screening project and signing this form does not obligate or commit me personally to participate in any other study or demonstration.

TO THE BEST OF MY KNOWLEDGE [ ] I AM NOT [ ] I AM [ ] I MAY BE   PREGNANT

X-ray mammography will not be performed on women who are or may be pregnant.

It is my intent to continue to participate in the program for the full period. I understand, however, that I may withdraw from the program at any time without prejudice or penalty.

[ ] I understand that I am eligible under the criteria for screening in Part II and wish to accept the mammographic examination.

[ ] I understand that I am eligible under criteria for screening in Part II but do not wish to accept the mammographic examination.

[ ] I understand that I am not eligible for mammography under the criteria for screening in Part II.

SIGNATURE (Screenee)   Date   Birthdate

Signature of Person Responsible
for Securing Informed Consent

DEPARTMENT OF HEALTH, EDUCATION, AND WELFARE
PUBLIC HEALTH SERVICE

NATIONAL INSTITUTES OF HEALTH
NATIONAL CANCER INSTITUTE — AMERICAN CANCER SOCIETY
BREAST CANCER DETECTION DEMONSTRATION PROJECT

NAME AND ADDRESS RECORD

1. OFFICE
(01-02)

2. ACCESSION NUMBER
(03-08)

3. FORM TYPE
(09-10)   1 1

4. EXAM NUMBER
(11-12)

FORM APPROVED
O.M.B. No. 68-R1377

ANNUAL SERIES   VISIT NUMBER

TO ENSURE THAT OUR RECORDS REFLECT YOUR CORRECT AND COMPLETE STATUS, PLEASE RESTATE IN FULL THE INFORMATION REQUESTED BELOW

5. PATIENT SIGNATURE   DATE

TWO INDIVIDUALS WITH WHOM I DO NOT RESIDE, THROUGH WHOM I MAY BE REACHED, OR WHO MAY BE CONTACTED ARE:

6. NAME   PHONE (Include Area Code)

ADDRESS (Include ZIP)

7. NAME   PHONE (Include Area Code)

ADDRESS (Include ZIP)

8. MY PERSONAL PHYSICIAN'S NAME IS   PHONE (Include Area Code)

9. ADDRESS (Include ZIP)

TO BE COMPLETED BY OFFICE PERSONNEL

10. NAME   LAST (13-27)   FIRST (28-37)   MIDDLE INITIAL (38)

11. ADDRESS (39-58)

12. CITY (59-71)   13. STATE (72-73)   14. ZIP CODE (74-78)

15. CENSUS TRACT (79-86)   16. DATE OF COMPLETION (87-92)   MONTH   DAY   YEAR

17. TELEPHONE (HOME)   AREA CODE   NUMBER   18. TELEPHONE (WORK)   AREA CODE   NUMBER

BREAST CANCER SCREENING PROGRAM
PATIENT HISTORY RECORD

TO BE FILLED OUT AT THE TIME OF EXAMINATION

1. OFFICE (01–02)

FORM APPROVED
O.M.B. NO. 68–R1377

2. ACCESSION NUMBER (03–08)

3. FORM TYPE (09–10)   `0` `2`

4. EXAM NUMBER (11–12)

Please read each question carefully to the patient. For questions that require coded answers, choose the code number that represents the patient's response and enter it in the box to the right of the question. Where the date is requested use the last two digits of the year, i.e. 1973 - ☐☐☐ . If the date is uncertain, record the patient's best recollection. DO NOT WRITE IN THE SHADED BOXES.

SECTION I — REASONS FOR EXAMINATION

WHY DID YOU ENTER THE BREAST CANCER
SCREENING PROGRAM
(Code: 1 — if the answer applies, otherwise leave blank.)

5. FOR ROUTINE CHECKUP ☐ (13)

6. I THOUGHT I MIGHT HAVE BREAST DISEASE ☐ (14)

7. I THOUGHT I MIGHT HAVE BREAST CANCER ☐ (15)

8. THERE IS A FAMILY HISTORY OF BREAST CANCER ☐ (16)

9. MY PHYSICIAN TOLD ME SOMETHING NEEDED CHECKING ☐ (17)

10. OTHER (Specify) _____ ☐ (18)

HOW DID YOU HEAR ABOUT THE PROGRAM
(Code: 1 - if the answer applies, otherwise leave blank)

11. TV ☐ (19)   16. MEETING (e.g., Women's Club) ☐ (24)

12. RADIO ☐ (20)   17. A FRIEND TOLD ME ☐ (25)

13. NEWSPAPER ☐ (21)   18. I was contacted by an American Cancer Society worker ☐ (26)

14. POSTER ☐ (22)   19. A PHYSICIAN ☐ (27)

15. CHURCH ☐ (23)   20. OTHER (Specify) ☐ (28)
_____

SECTION II — DEMOGRAPHIC DATA

21. WHAT IS YOUR RACE (Enter code number) ☐ (29)
   0 — Caucasian (White), not of Spanish origin
   1 — Caucasian (White), Spanish origin
   2 — Black, not of Spanish origin
   3 — Black, Spanish origin
   4 — American Indian/Eskimo
   5 — Japanese
   6 — Chinese
   7 — Other Oriental
   8 — Other (Specify) _____
   9 — Uncertain

22. WHAT IS YOUR RELIGION (Enter code number) ☐ (30)
   1 — Catholic
   2 — Jewish
   3 — Mormon
   4 — 7th Day Adventist
   5 — Protestant, other than Mormon or 7th Day Adventist
   6 — Other (Specify) _____
   7 — Uncertain
   8 — None

23. WHAT IS YOUR MARITAL STATUS ☐ (31)
   1 — Married   4 — Separated
   2 — Single   5 — Widowed
   3 — Divorced

24. WHEN WERE YOU BORN _____
   Month   Day   Year
   (FOR OFFICE USE ONLY)   (32–37)
   MONTH   DAY   YEAR

25. WHERE WERE YOU BORN

   If in U.S., Specify State _____

   If other country, specify _____

   (FOR OFFICE USE ONLY)   (38–39)

26. IN WHAT TYPE OF COMMUNITY WERE YOU BORN (Enter code number) ☐ (40)
   1 - Urban (population over 100,000)
   2 - Suburban (between 10,000–100,000)
   3 - Small town (population less than 10,000)
   4 - Rural (R.D. or R.R. #, farm)
   5 - Uncertain

27. WHERE WAS YOUR PREDOMINANT RESIDENCE AGE 10–20

   If in U.S. specify State _____

   If other country, specify_____

   (FOR OFFICE USE ONLY)   (41–42)

28. IN WHAT TYPE OF COMMUNITY WAS YOUR PREDOMINANT RESIDENCE AGE 10–20 ☐ (43)
   (Enter code number)
   1 - Urban (population over 100,000)
   2 - Suburban (between 10,000–100,000)
   3 - Small town (population less than 10,000)
   4 - Rural (R.D. or R.R.#, farm)
   5 - Uncertain

29. WHERE IS YOUR PRESENT RESIDENCE

   If in U.S., specify state _____

   If other country, specify_____

   (FOR OFFICE USE ONLY)   (44–45)

30. WHAT WAS YOUR TOTAL FAMILY INCOME LAST YEAR (Enter code number) ☐ (46)
   1 - Under   - $ 5,000
   2 - $ 5,000 - $ 9,999
   3 - $10,000 - $14,999
   4 - $15,000 - $29,999
   5 - $30,000 - $99,999
   6 - $100,000 and over
   7 - Uncertain

31. HOW MANY PEOPLE ARE SUPPORTED BY THIS INCOME (Enter number of people including yourself) ☐☐ (47–48)
   01   02   03   04   05   06   07   08   09   10   11   etc.

PATIENT HISTORY RECORD	OFFICE			ACCESSION NUMBER					

SECTION II - DEMOGRAPHIC DATA (continued)

32. WHAT WAS THE HIGHEST LEVEL OF GRADE SCHOOL EDUCATION YOU COMPLETED (Enter grade in school including high school)
01 02 03 04 05 06 07 08 09 10 11 12 ☐☐ (49-50)

33. POST HIGH SCHOOL (Enter number of years you completed in secretarial, business, beauty, or trade school, etc., where no college degree is involved.) ☐ (51)

34. JUNIOR COLLEGE AND COLLEGE (Enter number of years you completed) ☐ (52)

35. GRADUATE SCHOOL AND POST-GRADUATE WORK (Enter number of years you completed) ☐ (53)

36. WHAT WAS THE HIGHEST LEVEL OF EDUCATION COMPLETED BY YOUR (First) HUSBAND (Enter grade in school including high school. If uncertain, enter "99")
01 02 03 04 05 06 07 08 09 10 11 12 ☐☐ (54-55)

37. POST HIGH SCHOOL (Enter number of years your (first) husband completed in business or trade school, etc., where no college degree is involved. If uncertain, enter "9") ☐ (56)

38. JUNIOR COLLEGE AND COLLEGE (Enter number of years your (first) husband completed. If uncertain, enter "9") ☐ (57)

39. GRADUATE SCHOOL AND POST-GRADUATE WORK (Enter number of years your (first) husband completed. If uncertain, enter "9") ☐ (58)

SECTION III - FAMILY HISTORY OF CANCER (BLOOD RELATIVES ONLY)

40. HAVE ANY OF YOUR BLOOD RELATIVES LIVING OR DEAD (grandparents, parents, sisters, brothers, including half-sisters and half-brothers, sons, daughters, aunts or uncles only) EVER HAD CANCER ☐ (59)
1 - Yes
2 - No
3 - Uncertain
(If "No" enter "2" and skip to Question 65)

TO ANSWER QUESTIONS 41 THROUGH 46 USE THE FOLLOWING CODE:
1 - Yes
2 - No
3 - Uncertain

41. HAVE EITHER OF YOUR GRANDFATHERS EVER HAD CANCER ☐ (60)

42. HAVE EITHER OF YOUR GRANDMOTHERS EVER HAD CANCER (Other than breast) ☐ (61)

43. HAVE EITHER OF YOUR GRANDMOTHERS EVER HAD BREAST CANCER ☐ (62)

44. HAS YOUR FATHER EVER HAD CANCER ☐ (63)

45. HAS YOUR MOTHER EVER HAD CANCER (Other than breast) ☐ (64)

46. HAS YOUR MOTHER EVER HAD BREAST CANCER ☐ (65)

47. DO YOU HAVE A TWIN SISTER ☐ (66)
1 - Identical
2 - Fraternal
3 - No
4 - Uncertain
(If "No" enter "3" and skip to Question 50)

48. HAS YOUR TWIN SISTER EVER HAD CANCER (Other than breast) ☐ (67)
1 - Yes
2 - No
3 - Uncertain

49. HAS YOUR TWIN SISTER EVER HAD BREAST CANCER ☐ (68)
1 - Yes
2 - No
3 - Uncertain

TO ANSWER QUESTIONS 50 thru 64 enter the appropriate number in the boxes as follows. Include all relatives living or dead. 0 (none) 1 2 3 4 5 6 7 8 9 (or more)

50. HOW MANY SISTERS (other than twin) DO YOU HAVE OR HAVE YOU HAD ☐ (69)

51. HOW MANY DAUGHTERS ☐ (70)

52. HOW MANY AUNTS ☐ (71)

53. HOW MANY BROTHERS ☐ (72)

54. HOW MANY SONS ☐ (73)

55. HOW MANY UNCLES ☐ (74)

56. HOW MANY SISTERS (other than twin) HAVE EVER HAD CANCER (other than breast) ☐ (75)

57. HOW MANY DAUGHTERS HAVE EVER HAD CANCER (other than breast) ☐ (76)

58. HOW MANY AUNTS HAVE EVER HAD CANCER (other than breast) ☐ (77)

59. HOW MANY BROTHERS HAVE EVER HAD CANCER ☐ (78)

60. HOW MANY SONS HAVE EVER HAD CANCER ☐ (79)

61. HOW MANY UNCLES HAVE EVER HAD CANCER ☐ (80)

62. HOW MANY SISTERS (other than twin) HAVE EVER HAD BREAST CANCER ☐ (81)

63. HOW MANY DAUGHTERS HAVE EVER HAD BREAST CANCER ☐ (82)

64. HOW MANY AUNTS HAVE EVER HAD BREAST CANCER ☐ (83)

SECTION IV - BREAST DISEASE HISTORY

65. DO YOU NOW HAVE OR HAVE YOU EVER HAD AN INFECTION OF THE BREAST ☐ (84)
1 - Yes
2 - No
3 - Uncertain
(If "No" or "Uncertain", enter appropriate code and skip to Question 70)

IF "YES" GIVE LOCATION OF AFFECTED BREAST
1 - Right only
2 - Left only   NOW 66. ☐ (85)   PAST 67. ☐ (86)
3 - Both
4 - Uncertain

YEAR IT WAS FIRST NOTED   68. ☐☐ (87-88)   69. ☐☐ (89-90)

SECTION IV — BREAST DISEASE HISTORY (Continued)

70. DO YOU NOW HAVE OR HAVE YOU EVER HAD A LUMP OR CYST IN YOUR BREAST ☐ (91)
    1 - Yes
    2 - No
    3 - Uncertain
    (If "no" or "uncertain", enter appropriate code & skip to Question 75)

    IF "YES" GIVE LOCATION OF AFFECTED BREAST
    1 - Right only
    2 - Left only   NOW   PAST
    3 - Both   71. ☐   72. ☐
    4 - Uncertain   (92)   (93)

    YEAR IT WAS
    FIRST NOTED   73. ☐☐   74. ☐☐
                     (94-95)   (96-97)

75. DO YOU NOW HAVE OR HAVE YOU EVER HAD PAIN IN YOUR BREAST ☐ (98)
    1 - Yes
    2 - No
    3 - Uncertain
    (If "no" or "uncertain", enter appropriate code and skip to Question 80)

    IF "YES" GIVE LOCATION OF AFFECTED BREAST
    1 - Right only
    2 - Left only   NOW   PAST
    3 - Both   76. ☐   77. ☐
    4 - Uncertain   (99)   (100)

    YEAR IT WAS
    FIRST NOTED   78. ☐☐   79. ☐☐
                     (101-102)   (103-104)

80. DO YOU NOW HAVE OR HAVE YOU EVER HAD TENDERNESS IN YOUR BREAST ☐ (105)
    1 - Yes
    2 - No
    3 - Uncertain
    (If "no" or "uncertain", enter appropriate code and skip to Question 85)

    IF "YES" GIVE LOCATION OF AFFECTED BREAST
    1 - Right only
    2 - Left only   NOW   PAST
    3 - Both   81. ☐   82. ☐
    4 - Uncertain   (106)   (107)

    YEAR IT WAS
    FIRST NOTED   83. ☐☐   84. ☐☐
                     (108-109)   (110-111)

85. DO YOU NOW HAVE OR HAVE YOU EVER HAD SKIN CHANGES (color, wrinkles) IN YOUR BREAST ☐ (112)
    1 - Yes
    2 - No
    3 - Uncertain
    (If "no" or "uncertain", enter appropriate code and skip to Question 90)

    IF "YES" GIVE LOCATION OF AFFECTED BREAST
    1 - Right only
    2 - Left only   NOW   PAST
    3 - Both   86. ☐   87. ☐
    4 - Uncertain   (113)   (114)

    YEAR IT WAS
    FIRST NOTED   88. ☐☐   89. ☐☐
                     (115-116)   (117-118)

90. DO YOU NOW HAVE OR HAVE YOU EVER HAD A NON-BLOODY DISCHARGE (Fluid) FROM YOUR NIPPLE ☐ (119)
    1 - Yes
    2 - No
    3 - Uncertain
    (If "no" or "uncertain", enter appropriate code and skip to Question 95)

    IF "YES" GIVE LOCATION OF AFFECTED BREAST
    1 - Right only
    2 - Left only   NOW   PAST
    3 - Both   91. ☐   92. ☐
    4 - Uncertain   (120)   (121)

    YEAR IT WAS
    FIRST NOTED   93. ☐☐   94. ☐☐
                     (122-123)   (124-125)

95. DO YOU NOW HAVE OR HAVE YOU EVER HAD A BLOODY DISCHARGE (Fluid) FROM YOUR NIPPLE ☐ (126)
    1 - Yes
    2 - No
    3 - Uncertain
    (If "no" or "uncertain", enter appropriate code and skip to Question 100)

    IF "YES" GIVE LOCATION OF AFFECTED BREAST
    1 - Right only
    2 - Left only   NOW   PAST
    3 - Both   96. ☐   97. ☐
    4 - Uncertain   (127)   (128)

    YEAR IT WAS
    FIRST NOTED   98. ☐☐   99. ☐☐
                     (129-130)   (131-132)

100. DO YOU NOW HAVE OR HAVE YOU EVER HAD NIPPLE CHANGES IN THE BREAST ☐ (133)
    1 - Yes
    2 - No
    3 - Uncertain
    (If "no" or "uncertain", enter appropriate code and skip to Question 105)

    IF "YES" GIVE LOCATION OF AFFECTED BREAST
    1 - Right only
    2 - Left only   NOW   PAST
    3 - Both   101. ☐   102. ☐
    4 - Uncertain   (134)   (135)

    YEAR IT WAS
    FIRST NOTED   103. ☐☐   104. ☐☐
                     (136-137)   (138-139)

105. HAVE YOU EVER HAD TENDERNESS OF YOUR BREAST AT MENSTRUATION ☐ (140)
    1 - Never
    2 - In last 12 months
    3 - Before last 12 months
    4 - Uncertain
    (If "1", "2", or "4", skip to Question 107)

106. DATE OF ONSET (If before last 12 months) _____
                                                    Month   Year
         (FOR OFFICE USE ONLY) ░░░░░☐☐☐☐ (141-144)
                                       MONTH YEAR

107. HAVE YOU EVER HAD A NIPPLE DISCHARGE AT MENSTRUATION ☐ (145)
    1 - Never
    2 - In last 12 months
    3 - Before last 12 months
    4 - Uncertain
    (If "1", "2", or "4", skip to Question 109)

108. DATE OF ONSET (If before last 12 months) _____
                                                    Month   Year
         (FOR OFFICE USE ONLY) ░░░░░☐☐☐☐ (146-149)
                                       MONTH YEAR

PATIENT HISTORY RECORD	OFFICE			ACCESSION NUMBER					

SECTION IV — BREAST DISEASE HISTORY (Continued)

109. IF YOU NOW HAVE ANY SYMPTOMS, HAVE YOU SEEN A DOCTOR ☐ (150)
  1 - Yes
  2 - No

110. HAVE YOU EVER HAD BREAST SURGERY (Include biopsy) ☐ (151)
  1 - Yes, once
  2 - Yes, more than once
  3 - No
  4 - Uncertain
  (If "No" enter "3" and skip to Question 114)

111. IF "YES" GIVE LOCATION OF AFFECTED BREAST ☐ (152)
  1 - Right only
  2 - Left only
  3 - Both
  4 - Uncertain

112. YEAR IN WHICH FIRST BREAST SURGERY PERFORMED (If "Uncertain" enter "99") ☐ (153-154)
  YEAR

113. SURGICAL FINDINGS (results of surgery) ☐ (155)
  1 - Benign
  2 - Malignant
  3 - Uncertain

SECTION V — MEDICATION RECORD

Use the following code to answer next 7 questions
  1 - Now
  2 - Sometimes in the past but not now
  3 - Never
  4 - Uncertain

DO YOU NOW TAKE OR HAVE YOU TAKEN THE FOLLOWING

114. INSULIN ☐ (156)   **118.** FEMALE HORMONES ☐ (160)
  (Not birth control)

115. THYROID ☐ (157)   **119.** OTHER HORMONES ☐ (161)
  (Specify)

116. CORTISONE ☐ (158)   _____

117. ANTI-CANCER DRUGS (Specify) ☐ (159)   **120.** OTHER DRUGS (Specify) ☐ (162)

_____   _____

121. HAVE YOU EVER USED BIRTH CONTROL PILLS ☐ (163)
  1 - Now
  2 - Never
  3 - In the past
  4 - Uncertain
  (If "Never" enter "2" and skip to Question 128)

122. IF YOU DID WAS YOUR USE ☐ (164)
  1 - Continuous (regular)
  2 - Intermittent (not regular)

123. DO YOU REMEMBER WHEN YOU TOOK THE PILL ☐ (165)
  1 - Yes
  2 - No
  (If "No" enter "2" and skip to question 128)

124. IF "YES" WHAT WAS THE DATE YOU FIRST TOOK IT

  Month   Year
  (FOR OFFICE USE ONLY) ☐☐☐ (166-169)
  MONTH   YEAR

125. IF "YES" WHAT WAS THE DATE YOU LAST TOOK IT

  Month   Year
  (FOR OFFICE USE ONLY) ☐☐☐ (170-173)
  MONTH   YEAR

126. DO YOU REMEMBER HOW LONG YOU TOOK IT ☐ (174)
  1 - Yes
  2 - No
  (If "No" enter "2" and skip to question 128)

127. IF "YES" WHAT WAS TOTAL NUMBER OF YEARS AND/OR MONTHS YOU TOOK THE PILL

  Years   Months
  (FOR OFFICE USE ONLY) ☐☐☐ (175-176)
  YEARS   MONTHS

SECTION VI — SURGICAL AND RADIATION HISTORY

Use the following code to answer all questions in this section
  1 - Yes
  2 - No
  3 - Uncertain

128. HAVE YOU EVER HAD AN OPERATION FOR DISEASE OF YOUR UTERUS (Womb) OR OVARIES AT ANY TIME ☐ (179)
  (If "No" enter "2" and skip to Question 133)

129. IF "YES" HAS YOUR UTERUS (Womb) BEEN REMOVED ☐ (180)

130. WAS A SINGLE OVARY REMOVED AT ANY TIME ☐ (181)

131. WERE BOTH OVARIES REMOVED AT ANY TIME ☐ (182)

132. DID YOU STOP MENSTRUATING (having your periods) AFTER ONE OR BOTH OVARIES WERE REMOVED ☐ (183)

133. HAVE YOU EVER HAD X-RAY TREATMENT TO YOUR OVARIES OR UTERUS ☐ (184)

134. DID YOU STOP MENSTRUATING (having your periods) AFTER X-RAY TREATMENT ☐ (185)

135. HAVE YOU HAD X-RAY TREATMENT FOR ANY DISEASE OTHER THAN DISEASE OF THE OVARIES OR UTERUS ☐ (186)

SECTION VII — PREGNANCY HISTORY

136. WHAT IS YOUR PREGNANCY HISTORY ☐ (187)
  1 - Never pregnant
  2 - Not pregnant now but was in past
  3 - Pregnant within last year but not now
  4 - Pregnant now
  5 - Uncertain
  (If "Never" enter "1" or if "Uncertain" enter "5" and skip to Question 145.)

137. WHAT WAS YOUR AGE AT FIRST PREGNANCY - REGARDLESS OF OUTCOME. (Enter age in years) ☐☐ (188-189)

138. WHAT WAS YOUR AGE AT FIRST LIVE BIRTH (If "None" enter "99") ☐☐ (190-191)

SECTION VII — PREGNANCY HISTORY (Continued)

For the following questions enter the appropriate number in the box at the right

0 (none) 1 2 3 4 5 6 7 8 9 (or more)

139. HOW MANY LIVE BIRTHS HAVE YOU HAD ☐ (192)

140. HOW MANY STILLBIRTHS, ABORTIONS & MISCARRIAGES HAVE YOU HAD ☐ (193)

141. HOW MANY MONTHS WERE YOU PREGNANT IN YOUR FIRST PREGNANCY ☐ (194)

SECTION VIII — NURSING HISTORY

142. HOW MANY CHILDREN HAVE YOU BREAST-FED ☐ (195)
0 (none) 1 2 3 4 5 6 7 8 9 (or more)

143. HOW MANY TOTAL MONTHS OF BREAST-FEEDING (all children) HAVE YOU DONE

Number of months _____

(FOR OFFICE USE ONLY) ☐☐ (196-197)

144. IF YOU DID NOT BREAST-FEED YOUR CHILDREN, WHAT WAS THE REASON ☐ (198)
1 - Advised not to
2 - Did not wish to and never tried
3 - Unable to nurse, tried, but milk inadequate
4 - Other (Specify) _____

145. WERE YOU BREAST-FED AS A CHILD ☐ (199)
1 - Yes
2 - No
3 - Uncertain

SECTION IX - MENSTRUAL HISTORY

146. AT WHAT AGE DID YOUR MENSTRUAL PERIODS BEGIN ☐☐ (200-201)

147. IN COMPARISON WITH OTHER WOMEN DO YOU THINK THE AGE AT WHICH YOU STARTED HAVING PERIODS WAS (one of the following) ☐ (202)
1 - Normal
2 - Early
3 - Late
4 - Uncertain

148. HAVE YOUR PERIODS EVER BEEN IRREGULAR ☐ (203)
1 - Yes
2 - No
3 - Uncertain

149. HAVE YOU EVER BLED (Menstruated) MORE THAN 5 DAYS ☐ (204)
1 - Yes
2 - No
3 - Uncertain

150. HAS YOUR FLOW EVER BEEN EXCESSIVELY HEAVY AT TIMES ☐ (205)
1 - Yes
2 - No
3 - Uncertain

151. ARE YOU STILL HAVING PERIODS REGULARLY ☐ (206)
1 - Yes
2 - No
3 - Uncertain
(If "Yes" enter "1" & skip to Question 161.)

152. DID YOUR PERIODS STOP SUDDENLY ☐ (207)
1 - Yes
2 - No
3 - Uncertain

153. AT WHAT AGE DID YOUR PERIODS STOP ☐ (208-209)

154. WAS THE MENOPAUSE A DIFFICULT TIME ☐ (210)
1 - Yes
2 - No
3 - Somewhat
4 - Uncertain

155. DID YOU HAVE ANY HOT FLASHES OR FLUSHES ☐ (211)
1 - Yes
2 - No
3 - Uncertain

156. DID YOU SEE A DOCTOR ABOUT MENOPAUSE ☐ (212)
1 - Yes
2 - No
3 - Uncertain
(If "No" enter "2" and skip to Question 161.)

157. WAS MEDICINE PRESCRIBED ☐ (213)
1 - Yes
2 - No
3 - Uncertain

IF MEDICINE WAS PRESCRIBED, WAS IT ONE OF THE FOLLOWING

158. FEMALE HORMONE ☐ (214)
1 - Yes
2 - No
3 - Uncertain

159. MALE HORMONE ☐ (215)
1 - Yes
2 - No
3 - Uncertain

160. SEDATIVE ☐ (216)
1 - Yes
2 - No
3 - Uncertain

SECTION X — BREAST EXAMINATION HISTORY

161. HAVE YOU EVER EXAMINED YOUR BREASTS YOURSELF ☐ (217)
1 - Yes
2 - No

162. IF "NO" WHY NOT (Enter code number of the answer that most nearly applies and skip to Question 169.) ☐ (218)
1 - Don't want to
2 - Doctor checks instead
3 - Not much value
4 - Too much trouble
5 - Never thought of it
6 - Causes too much worry
7 - Don't know how
8 - Other (Specify) _____

163. IF "YES" WHEN DID YOU START _____
Month   Year
(FOR OFFICE USE ONLY) ☐☐☐☐ (219-222)

164. DO YOU STILL CHECK YOUR BREASTS ☐ (223)
1 - Yes
2 - No

PATIENT HISTORY RECORD	OFFICE			ACCESSION NUMBER					

SECTION X — BREAST EXAMINATION HISTORY (Continued)

165. IF "YES" HOW OFTEN
    1 - At least once a month
    2 - Once or twice a year
    3 - Uncertain   ☐ (224)

166. IF "NO" WHY DID YOU STOP
    1 - Don't want to anymore
    2 - Doctor checks instead
    3 - Not much value
    4 - Too much trouble
    5 - Never thought of it
    6 - Causes too much worry
    7 - Other (Specify)_____   ☐ (225)

167. WERE YOU TAUGHT TO EXAMINE YOUR BREASTS YOURSELF
    1 - Yes
    2 - No   ☐ (226)

168. IF "YES" INDICATE THE PRIMARY SOURCE OF INSTRUCTION
    1 - American Cancer Society
    2 - Personal physician
    3 - Medical clinic
    4 - Other (Specify)_____   ☐ (227)

169. HOW MANY TIMES HAS A DOCTOR EXAMINED YOUR BREASTS   ☐ (228)
    0 (never) 1 2 3 4 5 6 7 8 9 (or more)

170. IF YOU HAVE BEEN EXAMINED GIVE THE DATE OF THE LAST EXAMINATION
    Month   Year
    (FOR OFFICE USE ONLY) ☐☐☐☐ (229-232)

171. HOW MANY TIMES HAVE YOU BEEN CHECKED FOR BREAST CANCER BY X-RAY   ☐ (233)
    0 (never) 1 2 3 4 5 6 7 8 9 (or more)

172. IF YOU HAVE BEEN CHECKED BY X-RAY WHEN WAS IT LAST DONE _____
    Month   Year
    (FOR OFFICE USE ONLY) ☐☐☐.☐ (234-237)

SECTION XI — DISEASE HISTORY

Code for this entire Section (Questions 173—252)
    1 - Yes
    2 - No
    3 - Uncertain
    If "Yes" enter age at time of onset

173. HAVE YOU EVER HAD SERIOUS HAY FEVER, SKIN BLISTERS OR ITCHING DUE TO EATING OR TOUCHING CERTAIN FOOD, OR OTHER SUBSTANCES, OR SENSITIVITY TO PENICILLIN OR OTHER DRUGS   AGE ___ ☐ (238)

    (If "No" enter "2" and skip to Question 180.)

174. HAVE CERTAIN FOODS EVER UPSET YOU ___ ☐ (239)

175. HAVE YOU EVER DEVELOPED SKIN RASHES ___ ☐ (240)

176. HAVE DRUGS (penicillin, sedatives, etc.) EVER DISAGREED WITH YOU   AGE ___ ☐ (241)

177. HAVE YOU SNEEZED, ETC., FREQUENTLY FROM DUST, POLLEN, AND OTHER SUBSTANCES ___ ☐ (242)

178. HAVE YOU EVER WHEEZED OR HAD PROLONGED SHORTNESS OF BREATH (asthma) ___ ☐ (243)

179. OTHER ALLERGIES (Specify)_____ ☐ (244)

180. HAVE YOU EVER HAD ANY SERIOUS BLOOD DISEASE   AGE ___ ☐ (245)
    (If "No" enter "2" and skip to Question 186.)

181. ANEMIA ___ ☐ (246)

182. LEUKEMIA ___ ☐ (247)

183. SICKLE CELL DISEASE ___ ☐ (248)

184. POLYCYTHEMIA (too much blood) ___ ☐ (249)

185. OTHER SERIOUS BLOOD DISEASE (Specify)_____ ___ ☐ (250)

186. HAVE YOU EVER HAD SERIOUS TROUBLE WITH YOUR HEART OR BLOOD VESSELS (arteries and veins)   AGE ___ ☐ (251)
    (If "No" enter "2" and skip to Question 194.)

187. HYPERTENSION (high blood pressure) ___ ☐ (252)

188. ANGINA PECTORIS (chest pain during exercise) ___ ☐ (253)

189. MYOCARDIAL INFARCTION (heart attack) ___ ☐ (254)

190. THROMBOPHLEBITIS (milk leg, swollen leg) ___ ☐ (255)

191. RHEUMATIC FEVER (joint pain, St. Vitus Dance or high fever as a child or young adult.) ___ ☐ (256)

192. ARTERIOSCLEROSIS (hardened arteries with leg pain when you walk) ___ ☐ (257)

193. OTHER SERIOUS TROUBLE WITH HEART OR BLOOD VESSEL DISEASE ___ ☐ (258)

    (Specify) _____

PATIENT HISTORY RECORD	OFFICE			ACCESSION NUMBER					

SECTION XI — DISEASE HISTORY (Continued)
Code for Section XI is
1 - Yes
2 - No
3 - Uncertain
If "Yes" enter age at time of onset

AGE

194. HAVE YOU EVER HAD ABNORMAL FATNESS OR THINNESS, SUGAR IN YOUR URINE, UNUSUAL HAIR GROWTH, OR HAD YOUR SKIN BECOME UNUSUALLY DARK
(If "No" enter "2" and skip to Question 203.) (259)

195. DIABETES MELLITUS (sugar in urine) (260)

196. HYPOGLYCEMIA (too little sugar) (261)

197. HYPOADRENALISM (Addison's Disease) (262)

198. HYPOTHYROIDISM (too little thyroid) (263)

199. HYPERTHYROIDISM (too much thyroid) (264)

200. GOITER (swelling in throat) (265)

201. OSTEOPOROSES (soft bones) (266)

202. OTHER ENDOCRINE DISORDERS (Specify) _____ (267)

AGE

203. HAVE YOU EVER HAD SERIOUS OR PROLONGED SHORTNESS OF BREATH, COUGH, COUGHED UP BLOOD OR HAD SEVERE PAIN WITH BREATHING IN THE PAST OR RECENTLY
(If "No" enter "2" and skip to Question 208.) (268)

204. EMPHYSEMA (269)

205. PNEUMONIA (lung infection) (270)

206. TUBERCULOSIS OF LUNGS (271)

207. OTHER LUNG DISEASE (Specify) (272)
_____

AGE

208. HAVE YOU EVER HAD SEVERE PAINS OR TENDERNESS IN YOUR BONES, JOINTS OR BACK
(If "No" enter "2" and skip to Question 213.) (273)

209. RHEUMATISM (arthritis) (274)

AGE

210. BURSITIS (pain in shoulder or hips) (275)

211. OSTEOMYELITIS (infection of bones) (276)

212. OTHER MUSCULO-SKELETAL PROBLEMS (Specify) _____ (277)

AGE

213. HAVE YOU EVER HAD SERIOUS DISEASE OF YOUR BOWELS (gut) OR ABDOMEN (belly)
(If "No" enter "2" and skip to Question 221.) (278)

214. APPENDICITIS (gradual or sudden pain in abdomen) (279)

215. COLITIS (frequent, watery or bloody bowel movements) (280)

216. PERITONITIS (severe and serious abdominal pain) (281)

217. DIVERTICULITIS (intermittent pain in lower abdomen (282)

218. PANCREATITIS (severe upper abdominal (belly) pain with yellow jaundice (yellow skin)) (283)

219. INTESTINAL OBSTRUCTION (cannot move bowels and have severe abdominal pain - "bellyache") (284)

220. OTHER GASTRO-INTESTINAL DISEASE (Specify) _____ (285)
_____

AGE

221. HAVE YOU EVER HAD SERIOUS LIVER DISEASE
(If "No" enter "2" and skip to Question 227.) (286)

222. HEPATITIS (infection of the liver) (287)

223. CIRRHOSIS OF THE LIVER (288)

224. CHOLELITHIASIS (gallstones) (289)

225. CHOLECYSTITIS (infection of gall bladder) (290)

226. OTHER LIVER DISEASE (Specify) (291)
_____

| PATIENT HISTORY RECORD | OFFICE | | | ACCESSION NUMBER | | | | | |

SECTION XI — DISEASE HISTORY (Continued)
Code for Section XI is
1 - Yes
2 - No
3 - Uncertain
If "Yes" enter age at time of onset

AGE

227. HAVE YOU EVER HAD SERIOUS KIDNEY
OR BLADDER DISEASE _____ [ ] (292)
(If "No" enter "2" and skip to Question 232.)

228. NEPHROLITHIASIS (kidney stones) _____ [ ] (293)

229. BRIGHT'S DISEASE, NEPHRITIS _____ [ ] (294)
(kidney disease)

230. CYSTITIS (infection of the bladder) _____ [ ] (295)

231. OTHER URINARY DISEASE (Specify) _____ [ ] (296)

_____

AGE

232. HAVE YOU EVER HAD SERIOUS
DISEASE OF THE BRAIN OR NERVES _____ [ ] (297)
(If "No" enter "2" and skip to Question 239.)

233. EPILEPSY (fits or convulsions) _____ [ ] (298)

234. MENINGITIS _____ [ ] (299)

235. PARKINSON'S DISEASE (severe tremor _____ [ ] (300)
and difficulty walking)

236. STROKE, APOPLECTIC (paralysis due to _____ [ ] (301)
blood clot or hemorrhage)

237. ENCEPHALITIS (inflammation of brain) _____ [ ] (302)

238. OTHER DISEASE OF THE BRAIN OR _____ [ ] (303)
NERVES (Specify) _____

_____

AGE

239. HAVE YOU EVER HAD CANCER _____ [ ] (304)
(If "No" enter "2" and your interview is complete.)

240. SKIN CANCER _____ [ ] (305)

241. CERVICAL CANCER (uterine cervix) _____ [ ] (306)

242. ADENOMA OF UTERUS (uterine body) _____ [ ] (307)

243. CANCER OF UTERUS BUT DO NOT _____ [ ] (308)
KNOW WHICH KIND

AGE

244. BREAST _____ [ ] (309)

245. COLON (bowel) _____ [ ] (310)

246. OVARY _____ [ ] (311)

247. OTHER FORMS OF CANCER (Specify) _____ [ ] (312)

_____

AGE

248. IF YOU HAD CANCER WAS YOUR _____ [ ] (313)
CANCER TREATED
(If "No" enter "2" and your interview
is complete)

249. SURGERY _____ [ ] (314)

250. X-RAY _____ [ ] (315)

251. DRUGS _____ [ ] (316)

252. OTHER TREATMENT (Specify) _____ [ ] (317)

_____

(FOR OFFICE USE ONLY)

253. INTERVIEWER IDENTIFICATION [. .] (318–320)

254. DATE OF
INTERVIEW _____
MONTH DAY YEAR

[ ] (321–326)
MONTH DAY YEAR

255. COMMENTS

DEPARTMENT OF HEALTH, EDUCATION, AND WELFARE
PUBLIC HEALTH SERVICE
NATIONAL INSTITUTES OF HEALTH
NATIONAL CANCER INSTITUTE - AMERICAN CANCER SOCIETY

**BREAST CANCER DETECTION DEMONSTRATION PROJECT
RECALL PATIENT HISTORY RECORD**

FORM APPROVED
O.M.B. 68-R1377

1. OFFICE (01 02) ☐☐

2. ACCESSION NUMBER (03 08) ☐☐☐☐☐☐ ANNUAL SERIES ☐ VISIT NUMBEI

3. FORM TYPE (09 10) 1 2

4. EXAM NUMBER (11-12) ☐ --- ☐

INTERVIEWER INSTRUCTIONS. Please read each question carefully to the patient. For questions that require coded answers, choose the code number that represents the patient's response and enter it in the box to the right of the question. Where the date is requested use the last two digits of the year, i.e. 1973 — 7 3 If the date is uncertain, record the patient's best recollection. Code month as January - 01, February - 02, etc.

DATE OF LAST EXAM _____ _____ _____
MONTH   DAY   YEAR

5. WHAT IS YOUR MARITAL STATUS (Enter code) ☐ (13)
   1 - Married   4 - Separated
   2 - Single   5 - Widowed
   3 - Divorced

6. SINCE YOUR LAST EXAMINATION HERE, HAVE ANY OF YOUR FEMALE BLOOD RELATIVES ☐ (14)
(Grandmothers, Mother, Sisters - including half-sisters, daughters or aunts only) DEVELOPED BREAST CANCER
   1 - Yes
   2 - No
   3 - Uncertain

7. DO YOU NOW HAVE A BREAST INFECTION ☐ (15)
   1 - Yes
   2 - No
   3 - Uncertain

8. IF "YES", WHICH BREAST ☐ (16)
   1 - Right only   3 - Both
   2 - Left only   4 - Uncertain

9. DO YOU NOW HAVE A LUMP IN YOUR BREAST ☐ (17)
   1 - Yes
   2 - No
   3 - Uncertain

10. IF "YES", WHICH BREAST ☐ (18)
   1 - Right only   3 - Both
   2 - Left only   4 - Uncertain

11. SINCE YOUR LAST EXAMINATION HAVE YOU HAD A DISCHARGE (Fluid) FROM YOUR ☐ (19)
NIPPLE (Other than when you were pregnant or nursing a child)
   1 - Yes
   2 - No
   3 - Uncertain

12. IF "YES", WHICH BREAST ☐ (20)
   1 - Right only   3 - Both
   2 - Left only   4 - Uncertain

13. IF YOU NOW HAVE ANY OF THESE BREAST SYMPTOMS, HAVE YOU SEEN A DOCTOR ☐ (21)
   1 - Yes   3 - No symptoms present
   2 - No

14. SINCE YOUR LAST EXAMINATION HAVE YOU HAD BREAST SURGERY (Include a biopsy) ☐ (22)
   1 - Yes, once   3 - No
   2 - Yes, more than once 4 - Uncertain

   If "NO", enter "3" and skip to Question 18.

15. IF "YES", WHICH BREAST ☐ (23)
   1 - Right only   3 - Both
   2 - Left only   4 - Uncertain

16. DATE BREAST SURGERY WAS PERFORMED ☐☐ ☐☐ (24 27)
MONTH   YEAR

---

17. SURGICAL FINDINGS (Result of Surgery) ☐ (28)
   1 - Benign
   2 - Malignant
   3 - Uncertain

18. ARE YOU NOW TAKING BIRTH CONTROL PILLS ☐ (29)
   1 - Yes
   2 - No
   3 - Uncertain

19. ARE YOU NOW TAKING FEMALE HORMONES ☐ (30)
(Not birth control pills)
   1 - Yes
   2 - No
   3 - Uncertain

20. ARE YOU NOW PREGNANT ☐ (31)
   1 - Yes
   2 - No
   3 - Uncertain

21. WHEN WAS THE BEGIN-NING OF YOUR LAST MENSTRUAL PERIOD ☐☐ ☐☐ ☐☐ (32-37)
MONTH DAY YEAR
(Enter only the year if last menstrual period was more than 6 months ago)

22. SINCE YOUR LAST VISIT HERE, HAVE YOU EXAMINED YOUR BREASTS YOURSELF ☐ (38)
   1 - Yes but only a few times
     (History is completed)
   2 - Yes, Regularly
   3 - No

23. IF "NO", WHY NOT (Enter code number of the answer that most nearly applies) ☐ (39)
   1 - Don't want to
   2 - Doctor checks instead
   3 - Not much value
   4 - Too Much trouble
   5 - Never thought of it
   6 - Causes too much worry
   7 - Don't know how
   8 - Other (Specify)

24. IF "YES REGULARLY", HOW OFTEN DO YOU EXAMINE YOUR BREASTS ☐ (40)
   1 - A few times a year (1-3 times)
   2 - Several times a year (4-11 times)
   3 - At least once a month
   4 - Uncertain

FOR OFFICE USE ONLY

25. INTERVIEWER'S IDENTIFICATION ☐☐☐ (41 43)

26. DATE OF INTERVIEW ☐☐ ☐☐ ☐☐ (44 49)
MONTH DAY YEAR

COMMENTS

MICROFILM NO.

NATIONAL CANCER INSTITUTE—AMERICAN CANCER SOCIETY	1. OFFICE (01—02)
BREAST CANCER SCREENING PROGRAM	2. ACCESSION NUMBER (03—08)
THERMOGRAPHY RECORD	3. FORM TYPE (09—10) **0 5** 4. EXAM NUMBER (11—12)

FORM APPROVED
O.M.B. NO. 68—R1377

ANNUAL SERIES   VISIT NUMBER

Check (✓) the appropriate box unless otherwise indicated. Do not write in the shaded boxes.
Answer all questions, some may require multiple answers.

SECTION I — SYMMETRY

5. IS THERE SYMMETRY IN THE BACKGROUND TEMPERATURE OF THE TWO BREASTS

	YES	NO
ANTEROPOSTERIOR PROJECTION	1 (13-1)	2 (13-2)
OBLIQUE PROJECTION	1 (14-1)	2 (14-2)

6. IF ASYMMETRIC, INDICATE SIDE AND LOCATION OF INCREASED HEAT EMISSION

RIGHT		LEFT
(15) 1	BREAST ABSENT	1 (16)
(17) 1	UPPER OUTER QUANDRANT	1 (18)
(19) 1	UPPER INNER QUANDRANT	1 (20)
(21) 1	LOWER OUTER QUANDRANT	1 (22)
(23) 1	LOWER INNER QUANDRANT	1 (24)
(25) 1	CENTRAL	1 (26)
(27) 1	DIFFUSE	1 (28)

7. IS THERE APPROXIMATE SYMMETRY BETWEEN THE VASCULAR PATTERNS OF THE TWO BREASTS

	YES	NO
ANTEROPOSTERIOR PROJECTION	1 (29-1)	2 (29-2)
OBLIQUE PROJECTION	1 (30-1)	2 (30-2)

8. IF ASYMMETRIC, INDICATE LOCATION OF DISTORTION ASYMMETRY

RIGHT		LEFT
(31) 1	BREAST ABSENT	1 (32)
(33) 1	UPPER OUTER QUANDRANT	1 (34)
(35) 1	UPPER INNER QUANDRANT	1 (36)
(37) 1	LOWER OUTER QUANDRANT	1 (38)
(39) 1	LOWER INNER QUANDRANT	1 (40)
(41) 1	CENTRAL	1 (42)
(43) 1	DIFFUSE	1 (44)

9. DESCRIBE DISTORTION CAUSING ASYMMETRY

RIGHT		LEFT
(45) 1	INCREASED NUMBER OF VEINS	1 (46)
(47) 1	INCREASED CALIBER OF VEINS	1 (48)
(49) 1	INCREASED TEMPERATURE OF VEINS	1 (50)

SECTION II — THERMAL DESCRIPTION

10. IS THE OVERALL TEMPERATURE LEVEL OF THE TWO AREOLAE APPROXIMATELY EQUAL

	YES	NO
ANTEROPOSTERIOR PROJECTION	1 (51-1)	2 (51-2)
OBLIQUE PROJECTION	1 (52-1)	2 (52-2)

11. IF UNEQUAL INDICATE SIDE OF INCREASED HEAT EMISSION

RIGHT	LEFT
1 (53-1)	2 (53-2)

12. INDICATE ABSOLUTE TEMPERATURE DIFFERENCE (in °c) BETWEEN THE WARMEST AND COLDEST AREAS OF EACH BREAST AS DETERMINED BY ISOTHERM READINGS

RIGHT_____ . _____ °C   (54-55)

LEFT _____ . _____ °C   (56-57)

SECTION III — RECOMMENDATIONS

(Base your recommendations only on the thermography examination)

13. WHAT IS YOUR INTERPRETATION OF THE EXAMINATION

RIGHT		LEFT
(58-1) 1	RESULTS NEGATIVE	1 (59-1)
(58-2) 2	RESULTS ABNORMAL	2 (59-2)
(58-3) 3	TECHNICALLY UNSATISFACTORY	3 (59-3)

14. RE-EXAMINE BEFORE 12 MONTH RECALL

YES	NO
1 (60-1)	2 (60-2)

(61-62)

15. RE-EXAMINE IN _____ MONTHS
(If rescreening date to be determined later, enter "99")

16. EXPRESS YOUR CONFIDENCE LEVEL IN YOUR THERMOGRAPHIC IMPRESSION ON A 1 to 5 SCALE. (Circle appropriate number)

1   2   3   4   5   (63)

17. EQUIPMENT _____   (64-66)

18. EXAMINER IDENTIFICATION _____   (67-69)

19. DATE OF EXAMINATION _____

MONTH	DAY	YEAR

(70-75)

MONTH	DAY	YEAR

192

DEPARTMENT OF HEALTH, EDUCATION, AND WELFARE
PUBLIC HEALTH SERVICE
NATIONAL INSTITUTES OF HEALTH
NATIONAL CANCER INSTITUTE - AMERICAN CANCER SOCIETY
BREAST CANCER DETECTION DEMONSTRATION PROJECT

MAMMOGRAPHY RECORD

FORM APPROVED
O.M.B. NO. 68-R1377

1. OFFICE (01-02)
2. ACCESSION NUMBER (03-08)
   ANNUAL SERIES | VISIT NUMBER
3. FORM TYPE (09-10) | 0 | 4 |
4. EXAM NUMBER (11-12)

Circle the appropriate box unless otherwise indicated.
Answer all questions unless otherwise indicated; some may require multiple answers.

SECTION I – PHYSICAL DESCRIPTION

5. MEASURE THE MAXIMUM ANTEROPOSTERIOR DIAMETER OF THE BREASTS IN THE CEPHALOCAUDAD VIEW IN CM.

RIGHT (13-15)   LEFT (16-18)

6. DESCRIBE THE GENERAL CHARACTERISTICS OF THE BREAST TISSUE (Circle all that apply).

RIGHT		LEFT
(19) 1	ATROPHIC OR FATTY	1 (20)
(21) 2	INTERMEDIATE	2 (22)
(23) 3	GLANDULAR	3 (24)
(25) 4	HOMOGENEOUSLY DENSE	4 (26)

7. WHAT IS THE DUCTAL PATTERN? (CIRCLE ALL THAT APPLY)

RIGHT		LEFT
(27) 1	NORMAL	1 (28)
(29) 2	SUBAREOLAR THICKENING	2 (30)
(31) 3	DILATATION	3 (32)
(33) 4	DISTORTED OR IRREGULAR	4 (34)

8. ARE THE GLANDULAR PATTERNS OF THE BREASTS SYMMETRICAL? (BLANK IF EXAM DONE ON ONLY ONE SIDE)

YES 1 (35-1)

NO 2 (35-2)

9. IS THERE SKIN THICKENING? (CIRCLE ALL THAT APPLY)

RIGHT		LEFT
(36) 1	NONE	1 (37)
(38) 2	LOCALIZED	2 (39)
(40) 3	AREOLAR	3 (41)
(42) 4	DIFFUSE	4 (43)
(44) 5	RETRACTION	5 (45)

COMMENTS:

_____
_____
_____
_____
_____
_____

10. ARE THERE NIPPLE CHANGES?

RIGHT		LEFT
(46-1) 1	NONE	1 (47-1)
(46-2) 2	RETRACTION	2 (47-2)
(46-3) 3	ENLARGEMENT	3 (47-3)
(46-4) 4	NOT VISUALIZED	4 (47-4)

11. ARE THERE LOCALIZED AREAS OF DISTORTED BREAST ARCHITECTURE OR NON-SPECIFIC INCREASES IN DENSITY?

RIGHT		LEFT
(48-1) 1	YES, LOCALIZED	1 (49-1)
(48-2) 2	YES, DIFFUSE	2 (49-2)
(48-3) 3	NO	3 (49-3)

12. IF "YES", CIRCLE THE LOCATIONS OF THE CENTERS OF SUCH AREAS (CIRCLE ALL THAT APPLY).

RIGHT		LEFT
(50) 1	UPPER OUTER	1 (51)
(52) 2	UPPER INNER	2 (53)
(54) 3	LOWER OUTER	3 (55)
(56) 4	LOWER INNER	4 (57)
(58) 5	CENTRAL	5 (59)
(60) 6	DIFFUSE	6 (61)

13. DOES THE PATIENT HAVE A PREVIOUS MAMMOGRAM?

RIGHT		LEFT
(62-1) 1	YES	1 (63-1)
(62-2) 2	NO	2 (63-2)

14. IF "YES", HAS THERE BEEN A SIGNIFICANT CHANGE?

RIGHT		LEFT
(64-1) 1	YES	1 (65-1)
(64-2) 2	NO	2 (65-2)

SECTION II – PATHOLOGY

15. ARE THERE MASSES PRESENT IN ONE OR BOTH BREASTS?

RIGHT		LEFT
(66-1) 1	NONE	1 (67-1)
(66-2) 2	1 MASS	2 (67-2)
(66-3) 3	2 MASSES	3 (67-3)
(66-4) 4	3 OR MORE MASSES	4 (67-4)

IF "NONE" FOR BOTH BREASTS SKIP TO QUESTION 21.

MAMMOGRAPHY RECORD	OFFICE			ACCESSION NUMBER					

SECTION II – PATHOLOGY (continued)

16. WHERE ARE THE MASSES LOCATED? (CIRCLE LOCATION OF THE CENTER OF EACH MASS.)

RIGHT				LEFT		
1ST (CIRCLE ONLY ONE BOX)	2ND (CIRCLE ONLY ONE BOX)	MULTIPLE (CIRCLE ALL THAT APPLY)		1ST (CIRCLE ONLY ONE BOX)	2ND (CIRCLE ONLY ONE BOX)	MULTIPLE (CIRCLE ALL THAT APPLY)
(68)	1 (69)	1 (70)	DIFFUSE	1 (80)	1 (81)	1 (82)
2	2	2 (71)	UPPER OUTER	2	2	2 (83)
3	3	3 (72)	LOWER OUTER	3	3	3 (84)
4	4	4 (73)	UPPER INNER	4	4	4 (85)
5	5	5 (74)	LOWER INNER	5	5	5 (86)
6	6	6 (75)	AREOLAR	6	6	6 (87)
7	7	7 (76)	UPPER PARASTERNAL	7	7	7 (88)
8	8	8 (77)	LOWER PARASTERNAL	8	8	8 (89)
9	9	9 (78)	AXILLARY PROLONGATION	9	9	9 (90)
0	0	0 (79)	CENTRAL	0	0	0 (91)

17. WHAT ARE THE IMAGING CHARACTERISTICS OF EACH MASS? (CIRCLE THE MOST APPROPRIATE CHARACTERISTIC)

RIGHT				LEFT		
1ST	2ND	MULTIPLE		1ST	2ND	MULTIPLE
1 (92–1)	1 (93–1)	1 (94)	PARTIALLY IMAGED	1 (96–1)	1 (97–1)	1 (98)
2 (92–2)	2 (93–2)	2 (95)	COMPLETELY IMAGED	2 (96–2)	2 (97–2)	2 (99)

18. WHAT ARE THE MARGINAL CHARACTERISTICS OF EACH MASS? (CIRCLE THE MOST APPROPRIATE CHARACTERISTIC)

RIGHT				LEFT		
1ST	2ND	MULTIPLE		1ST	2ND	MULTIPLE
1 (100–1)	1 (101–1)	1 (102)	ILL-DEFINED	1 (104–1)	1 (105–1)	1 (106)
2 (100–2)	2 (101–2)	2 (103)	WELL-DEFINED	2 (104–2)	2 (105–2)	2 (107)

19. WHAT IS THE SHAPE OF EACH MASS? (CHECK THE MOST APPROPRIATE DESCRIPTION)

RIGHT				LEFT		
1ST	2ND	MULTIPLE		1ST	2ND	MULTIPLE
(108) 1	(109) 1	1 (110)	OVAL OR ROUND	(115) 1	(116) 1	1 (117)
2	2	2 (111)	MULTINODULAR	2	2	2 (118)
3	3	3 (112)	STELLATE OR SPICULATED	3	3	3 (119)
4	4	4 (113)	COMBINATION OF ABOVE	4	4	4 (120)
5	5	5 (114)	OTHER (SPECIFY)	5	5	5 (121)

20. MEASURE IN MILLIMETERS THE GREATEST DIAMETER(S) OF THE SUSPECT MASS OR MASSES

RIGHT			LEFT	
1ST	2ND		1ST	2ND
mm (122–123)	mm (124–125)	A.P. (CEPHALOCAUDAD VIEW)	mm (134–135)	mm (136–137)
mm (126–127)	mm (128–129)	TRANSVERSE (CEPHALOCAUDAD VIEW)	mm (13?–139)	mm (140–141)
mm (130–131)	mm (132–133)	VERTICAL (OBLIQUE VIEW)	mm (142–143)	mm (144–145)

MAMMOGRAPHY RECORD	OFFICE		ACCESSION NUMBER					

SECTION II – PATHOLOGY (continued)

21. DESCRIBE THE NON-VASCULAR CALCIFICATIONS.

RIGHT		(CIRCLE ALL THAT APPLY)		LEFT
(146)	1	NONE	1	(147)
(148)	2	PUNCTATE	2	(149)
(150)	3	RING-SHAPED	3	(151)
(152)	4	LINEAR	4	(153)
(154)	5	LARGE, CONGLOMERATE	5	(155)

22. WHAT IS THE DISTRIBUTION OF THE CALCIUM?

RIGHT		(CIRCLE ALL THAT APPLY)		LEFT
(156)	1	SINGLE	1	(157)
(158)	2	MULTIPLE	2	(159)
(160)	3	SCATTERED	3	(161)
(162)	4	LINEAR	4	(163)
(164)	5	CLUSTERED	5	(165)

23. IS THERE VEIN ENLARGEMENT? (IF NONE FOR BOTH BREASTS, SKIP TO QUESTION 26.)

RIGHT				LEFT
(166–1)	1	NONE	1	(167–1)
(166–2)	2	DIFFUSELY ENLARGED	2	(167–2)
(166–3)	3	FOCAL ENLARGEMENT	3	(167–3)

24. MEASURE IN MILLIMETERS THE DIAMETER OF THE LARGEST VEIN IN THE SUSPECT BREAST AND THEN THE DIAMETER OF THE CORRESPONDING VEIN IN THE OPPOSITE BREAST.

RIGHT		LEFT	
(168–169)	mm	(170–171)	mm

25. IF MEASUREMENT CANNOT BE MADE, INDICATE THE REASON.

RIGHT				LEFT
(172–1)	1	NOT MEASURABLE	1	(173–1)
(172–2)	2	NOT VISUALIZED	2	(173–2)

26. WHAT SIZE ARE THE VISUALIZED LYMPH NODES?

RIGHT				LEFT
(174)	1	NOT FILMED	1	(175)
(176)	2	NOT VISUALIZED	2	(177)
(178)	3	1.5 cm. OR LESS	3	(179)
(180)	4	OVER 1.5 cm.	4	(181)
(182)	5	FATTY INFILTRATION WITH ABOVE	5	(183)

27. HOW MANY LYMPH NODES ARE SEEN?

RIGHT		LEFT	
(184–185)			(186–187)

36. COMMENTS:

_____
_____
_____
_____

SECTION III – RECOMMENDATIONS

(BASE YOUR RECOMMENDATIONS ONLY ON THE MAMMOGRAPHY EXAMINATION.)

28. WHAT IS YOUR INTERPRETATION OF THE EXAMINATION?

RIGHT				LEFT
(188–189)	0 1	BREAST NORMAL	0 1	(190–191)
	0 2	TECHNICALLY UNSATISFACTORY EXAM	0 2	
	0 3	MASS OR MASSES PRESENT PROBABLY BENIGN	0 3	
	0 4	CALCIFICATION–NOT SUGGESTIVE OF MALIGNANCY	0 4	
	0 5	INCREASED DENSITY(IES) SUGGESTIVE OF MAMMARY DYSPLASIA	0 5	
	0 6	SINGLE MASS PRESENT – SUSPICION OF MALIGNANCY	0 6	
	0 7	MULTIPLE MASSES PRESENT – SUSPICION OF MALIGNANCY	0 7	
	0 8	SINGLE OR MULTIPLE MASSES PRESENT – CARCINOMA	0 8	
	0 9	ARCHITECTURAL DISTORTION – SUSPICION OF MALIGNANCY	0 9	
	1 0	CALCIFICATION – SUGGESTIVE OF MALIGNANCY	1 0	
	1 1	INCREASED DENSITY(IES) SUSPICION OF MALIGNANCY	1 1	
	1 2	BREAST REMOVED	1 2	
	1 3	EXAMINATION OMITTED	1 3	

29. RE-EXAMINE BEFORE 12-MONTH RECALL.

YES 1 (192–1)   NO 2 (192–2)

30. RE-EXAMINE IN_____MONTHS (193–194)
(IF RESCREENING DATE TO BE DETERMINED LATER, ENTER "99".)

31. TISSUE BIOPSY THE FOLLOWING (CIRCLE ALL THAT APPLY)

RIGHT				LEFT
(195)	1	NONE	1	(196)
(197)	2	MASS 1	2	(198)
(199)	3	MASS 2	3	(200)
(201)	4	ARCHITECTURAL DISTORTION	4	(202)
(203)	5	CALCIFICATIONS	5	(204)
(205)	6	OTHER (SPECIFY)	6	(206)

32. ASPIRATION IS RECOMMENDED (CIRCLE APPLICABLE BOX).

RIGHT 1 (207)   LEFT 2 (208)

33. TYPE OF EQUIPMENT. (209–211)

34. EXAMINER'S IDENTIFICATION. (212–214)

35. DATE OF EXAMINATION. MO DY YR (215–220)

37. EXPRESS YOUR CONFIDENCE LEVEL IN YOUR MAMMOGRAPHIC IMPRESSION ON A 1 TO 5 SCALE (CIRCLE APPROPRIATE NUMBER. OPTIONAL FOR LOCAL USE.)

1	2	3	4	5
Least				Most

DEPARTMENT OF HEALTH, EDUCATION, AND WELFARE
PUBLIC HEALTH SERVICE
NATIONAL INSTITUTES OF HEALTH
NATIONAL CANCER INSTITUTE - AMERICAN CANCER SOCIETY

BREAST CANCER DETECTION DEMONSTRATION PROJECT

PHYSICAL EXAMINATION RECORD

FORM APPROVED
O.M.B. NO. 68-R1377

1. OFFICE (01-02)

2. ACCESSION NUMBER (03-08)

3. FORM TYPE (09-10)   0   3

4. EXAM NUMBER (11-12)

ANNUAL SERIES   VISIT NUMBER

SECTION I – PHYSICAL DESCRIPTION

5. HEIGHT (inches) _____ (13-14)

6. WEIGHT (pounds) _____ (15-17)

7. IS THERE A BREAST ABSENT?
   1 – Yes   2 – No
   RIGHT (18)   LEFT (19)

8. BREAST SIZE
   1 – Small (AA, A)   2 – Medium (B, C)
   3 – Large (D or larger)   (20)

SECTION II – PATHOLOGY

9. IS THERE A MASS PRESENT? (If "None" for both breasts enter "1" and skip to question 21)

   1 – None
   2 – Single
   3 – Multiple
   4 – Diffuse

   RIGHT (21)   LEFT (22)

GIVE LOCATION OF EACH LESION OR ABNORMALITY. (Mark an "M" or "A" on the diagram below to indicate the Center of each mass or abnormality on both lateral and frontal views).

RIGHT LATERAL   RIGHT FRONTAL   LEFT FRONTAL   LEFT LATERAL

For each lesion marked with an "M" or an "A" in the above diagram, place the associated location code number in the appropriate box shown below.

	RIGHT			LESION	LEFT		
	LATERAL	FRONTAL	TYPE		FRONTAL	LATERAL	TYPE
10.	(23)	(24)	(25)	DOMINANT	(26)	(27)	(28)
11.	(29)	(30)	(31)	SECOND	(32)	(33)	(34)
12.	(35)	(36)	(37)	THIRD	(38)	(39)	(40)
13.	(41)	(42)	(43)	FOURTH	(44)	(45)	(46)

GIVE THE DIAMETER OF THE LARGEST DIMENSION (in centimeters) FOR EACH MASS PRESENT AND/OR ABNORMALITY.

	RIGHT		LEFT
14.	(47-48)	DOMINANT MASS	(49-50)
15.	(51-52)	SECOND	(53-54)
16.	(55-56)	THIRD	(57-58)
17.	(59-60)	FOURTH	(61-62)

GIVE DESCRIPTION OF THE DOMINANT MASS.

18. TEXTURE	19. MOBILITY	20. SHAPE
1 - Hard	1 - Moveable	1 - Discrete, regular
2 - Soft	2 - Fixed skin	2 - Irregular
3 - Cystic	3 - Fixed deep	

RIGHT	LEFT	RIGHT	LEFT	RIGHT	LEFT
(63)	(64)	(65)	(66)	(67)	(68)

SECTION III – OTHER CLINICAL DESCRIPTION

21. IS BREAST NODULARITY PRESENT? (To answer next four questions, use 1-Yes 2 - No)

   1 – None
   2 – Small
   3 – Large

   RIGHT (69)   LEFT (70)

22. IS BREAST THICKENING PRESENT?

   1 – None
   2 – Diffuse
   3 – Localized

   RIGHT (71)   LEFT (72)

23. (73) ARE THERE NIPPLE CHANGES? (74)

24. (75) ARE THERE SKIN CHANGES? (76)

25. (77) ARE THE AXILLARY NODES PALPABLE? (78)

26. (79) ARE THERE SIGNS OF RETRACTION? (80)

27. WHAT IS YOUR IMPRESSION OF THE EXAMINATION? (Circle Appropriate Box)

RIGHT (81)   LEFT (82)

1	NO MASS PRESENT
2	MASS OR MASSES PRESENT PROBABLY BENIGN
3	MASS OR MASSES PRESENT-SUSPICION OF MALIGNANCY
4	EXAMINATION OMITTED
5	BREAST REMOVED
6	BREAST DISEASE-PROBABLY BENIGN
7	BREAST DISEASE-SUSPICION OF MALIGNANCY

SECTION IV – RECOMMENDATIONS

28. RE-EXAMINE BEFORE 12-MONTH RECALL.
   1 - Yes   2 - No   (83)

29. RE-EXAMINE IN _____ MONTHS.
   (If rescreening date to be determined later, enter "99")   (84-85)

30. TISSUE BIOPSY
   RIGHT (86)   LEFT (87)
   1 - Yes   2 - No

31. ASPIRATION OF FLUID
   RIGHT (88)   LEFT (89)
   1 - Yes   2 - No

32. EXAMINER'S IDENTIFICATION   (90-92)

33. DATE OF EXAMINATION   MO   DY   YR   (93-98)

34. EXPRESS YOUR CONFIDENCE LEVEL IN YOUR PHYSICAL EXAM IMPRESSION ON A 1 to 5 SCALE. (Optional for local use. Circle appropriate number.)
   LEAST   1   2   3   4   5   MOST

DEPARTMENT OF HEALTH, EDUCATION, AND WELFARE
PUBLIC HEALTH SERVICE, NATIONAL INSTITUTES OF HEALTH
NATIONAL CANCER INSTITUTE — AMERICAN CANCER SOCIETY

BREAST CANCER DETECTION DEMONSTRATION PROJECT

FINAL SCREENING RECOMMENDATION

Form Approved
O.M.B. NO. 68-R1377

1. OFFICE (01-02)

2. ACCESSION NUMBER (03-08)

ANNUAL SERIES   VISIT NUMBER

3. FORM TYPE (09-10) **0 6**

4. EXAM NUMBER (11—12) - - -

Circle (o) the appropriate number in each question

Transcribe examination results exactly as recorded on the associated forms.

5. Has the Project made a previous recommendation for diagnostic surgery?

Yes No.
1   2
(13-1) (13-2)

6. Indicate reason for screening

1 = Initial   2 = Rescreen
3 = Medical Recall   4 = Technical Recall

(14)

SECTION I — FINDINGS

7. MAMMOGRAPHY EXAMINATION

Right
(15-16)

Left
(17-18)

01=Breast Normal
02=Technically Unsatisfactory
03=Mass or Masses Present-
Probably Benign
04=Calcification - Not Suggestive
of Malignancy
05=Increased Density(ies) - Suggestive of Mammary Dysplasia
06=Single Mass Present -
Suspicion of Malignancy
07=Multiple Masses Present -
Suspicion of Malignancy

08=Single or Multiple Masses
Present - Carcinoma
09=Architectural Distortion -
Suspicion of Malignancy
10=Calcification - Suggestive of
Malignancy
11=Increased Density(ies) -
Suspicion of Malignancy
12=Breast Removed
13=Examination Omitted
14=Examination Refused
15=Under 50, Not Recommended

8. Original Interpreter's Number
(19-21)

Right   Left

9. As a result of CORRELATION, I feel that
the interpretation should be:
(22-23)   (24-25)

10. PHYSICAL EXAMINATION

Right
(26)

Left
(27)

1 = No Mass Present
2 = Mass or Masses Present - Probably
Benign
3 = Mass or Masses Present - Suspicion
of Malignancy
4 = Examination Omitted
5 = Breast Removed
6 = Breast Disease - Probably Benign
7 = Breast Disease - Suspicion of
Malignancy

11. Original Examiner's Number
(28-30)

Right   Left

12. On RE-EXAMINATION, I feel that the
interpretation should be:
(31)   (32)

13. Re-Examiner's Number
(33-35)

14. THERMOGRAPHY EXAMINATION

Right

1 = Results Negative
2 = Results Abnormal
3 = Technically Unsatisfactory or
Incomplete
4 = Examination Omitted
5 = Breast Removed

(36)

Left
(37)

15. Original Interpreter's Number
(38-40)

16. As a result of CORRELATION, I feel that
the interpretation should be:

Right   Left
(41)   (42)

SECTION II — FINAL RECOMMENDATION

17. Is diagnostic surgery recommended?

Right   Left
(43) 1   NONE   2 (46)
(44) 3   BIOPSY   4 (47)
(45) 5   ASPIRATION 6 (48)

18. If there are BOTH Physical and
Mammographic abnormalities, are
they the same?   1 = Yes; 2 = No; 3 = Uncertain

(49)

19. On which modality was the diagnostic
surgery recommended?

1 = Physical; 2 = Mammogram; 3 = Both   (50)

20. (51-1) 1 Rescreen
(51-2) 2 Recall

in   months
(52-53)

21. (54-1) 1 Copied
(54-2) 2 Correlated

ID Number
(55-57)

22. Date of Screening

MO   DY   YR
(58-59) (60-61) (62-63)

23. Date of Completion

MO   DY   YR
(64-65) (66-67) (68-69)

24. 1 Circle if more than one significant finding on
(70) any modality

25. Comments:

Appendix B: Economic and Other Cost Considerations

John K. Gohagan

If this book were focused only on epidemiology and the technical capabilities of alternative detection modalities, there would be reason to introduce cost considerations into these discussions. However, selection among competing unimodality and multimodality screening protocols and the scheduling of examinations are our primary consideration. Since selection implies balancing potential benefits from action alternatives against competing costs (and risks), we have no alternative but to address the issues of cost estimation.

Each detection protocol has certain attendant costs. Some of the costs are of a direct financial nature, such as the cost of a mammogram, while others are psychosocial in nature, such as trauma associated with a false positive examination. In this appendix we discuss estimation problems and develop estimates that are used as starting points in the analytical chapters of the book. Dollar magnitudes for detection and treatment costs are estimated from local hospital data. Dollar magnitudes for other direct financial costs such as transportation are too small to have an impact on choices, so we do not estimate them. Dollar-equivalent values for psychosocial costs are estimated in terms or alternative market prices and

Surgical and biopsy data were compiled by Amy Hoffman, Department of Surgery, Barnes Hospital, and by Linda Beck, Department of Preventive Medicine at Washington University. Barnes Hospital, the two departments mentioned, and the Medical Care Group — a local health maintenance organization — cooperated in this effort. Early work in this area was done by Rita Menitoff. Laurie Tanen, a research assistant, worked on the problem of estimating psychosocial costs and valuing lives.

what economists call shadow prices. A dollar-equivalent value for the risk of radiation inherent in the use of mammography is estimated in terms of the potential for radiation-induced breast cancer. Dollar-equivalent values for a life lost are summarized from the literature in which they were estimated by three different and not completely satisfactory methods proposed by economists over the years.[1]

It would be nice if we could ignore the value of a human life in our analyses. But we cannot, for our attention is on individualized decision making, and the value of a life is a key parameter in the choice process. Since there is abundant evidence that humans view life as neither infinitely valuable nor of no value, we have no alternative but to establish reasonable bounds on the value of a human life if we are to proceed with analysis.

The cost estimates in this chapter are nothing more than that— estimates. They represent reasonable starting points for evaluation of choices. But extensive sensitivity studies are necessary to investigate the choice implications of variations from the starting estimates as a basis for final judgments on the relative merits of competing detection protocols. These sensitivity studies or analyses are accomplished in appropriate chapters as needed. Only the initial cost estimates are provided in this appendix.

PROCEDURAL COSTS

Procedural costs are the medical costs of detection, diagnosis, and treatment. In the detection process three modalities may be employed. These are clinical examination, mammography, and thermography.[2] Final diagnosis is accomplished via histological evaluation of a tissue sample.

Clinical examination may consist of brief questioning of a patient regarding previous breast problems in conjunction with palpation and visual inspection of the breast and axillary nodes by a nurse practitioner or a physician. But it may also include an extensive interview to develop a comprehensive family and personal medical history. The specific form of the examination varies depending on the practice. Also breast examination may constitute the primary reason for an office visit, or it may be only part of a general physical or gynecological examination. Hence, the cost of a clinical examination can vary substantially from visit to visit and from clinic to clinic. We treat clinical examination and extensive history taking as two distinct activities for the purpose of cost estimations.

Thermography and mammography are perhaps more precisely defined procedures, but charges for these modalities, too, vary substantially among clinics. Charges for these procedures cover materials, technician wages, equipment amortization, radiological interpretation, and frequently, marginal charges beyond the actual cost of doing the procedures.

Biopsy can mean many things. Usually, it refers to the surgical removal of all or part of a breast lesion for microscopic evaluation. This is how we use the term. The charges for a biopsy cover anesthetic and surgical services, operating room rent, medication, pathology, and hospital stay. In some cases a needle can be used to gather a tissue sample for evaluation. Needle biopsy is less expensive and less traumatic than surgical biopsy, but it is not common practice yet.

Treatment is a much more complex process than detection and diagnosis. Most of the charges are typical of, though larger than those for, excisional biopsy. But there are also charges for follow-up visits, adjuvant therapy, and possibly breast reconstruction. Furthermore, surgical procedures vary from removal of only the part of the breast containing the mass (segmental mastectomy) to removal of the entire breast (simple mastectomy) or to removal of the breast, the axillary lymph nodes, and perhaps muscle of the chest wall (radical mastectomy). Our cost estimates for surgery reflect this complexity.

Treatment of minimal cancers, tumors no larger than a centimeter in diameter with no nodal involvement, can be less severe than treatment of more advanced cancers. For example, segmental excision of small tumors, perhaps followed by radiation therapy, may be adequate for minimal cancers, while radical mastectomy followed by radiation and possibly chemotherapy is indicated for metastatic cancers. (See Chapter 11.) Also recurrence is more likely for cases first treated at later stages of development, as indicated in Table B.1. Consequently, treatment costs tend to increase with disease stage. And although one cannot determine the strength of this trend by statistical techniques from our data, one would expect a simple parametric relation like the following, with R representing a scaling factor to represent the situation adequately:

$$\begin{pmatrix} \text{Cost of Treatment} \\ \text{for} \\ \text{Advanced Cancer} \end{pmatrix} = (1 + R) \begin{pmatrix} \text{Cost of Treatment} \\ \text{for} \\ \text{Minimal Cancer} \end{pmatrix}$$

This formulation is quite useful for parametric analyses.

Tables B.2 and B.3 summarize our estimates of costs for detection, diagnosis, and treatment from records of Washington University-affiliated hospitals. Since there is a great deal of variability in cost data, we give ranges in lieu of individual values.

OTHER FINANCIAL COSTS

Periodic examinations take a woman away from her other activities for perhaps one-half day each time. Diagnostic biopsy, as distinguished from therapeutic surgery, can incapacitate a woman for two or three days.

TABLE B.1

Approximate Recurrence Rates for Breast Cancer by Disease Stage at Initial Treatment (in percent)

| Time (years) | Localized Disease | Metastatic Disease | |
		Regional	Systemic
5	20–30 (15)*	50–70 (34)	70–90 (59)
10	25–40 (22)	60–70 (48)	90–95 (72)
15	25–40	70–90	90–95
20	50–70	80–90	95–100

*Numbers in parenthesis are attributed to Perfler by Vorherr [1980]. These appear to represent a well-controlled and -monitored series.

Source: Based on survival data presented in Vorherr [1980].

Note: The great variability in these numbers represents the great variability in study populations and conditions.

Therapeutic surgery, recuperation, and follow-up can consume many weeks of time otherwise available for normal activities. And hospital or physician visits for adjuvant therapy, too, can consume weeks of time over the course of treatment.

Time spent in these activities could have been spent in other activities and must be valued at least at the level of alternative activities. If this time would have been spent in caring for a family, it must be worth at least as much as it would cost to hire a housekeeper to carry out the ordinary tasks of home management. Of course, families vary in size, needs, and circumstances, so one would expect considerable variation in estimates of such costs. For such services $5 to $10 per hour is not unreasonable.[3] Hence, an examination or follow-up visit might cost a woman $20 to $40 in time lost. Similar costs for a negative biopsy might be $120 to $360, assuming 12-hour working days for homemakers. For therapeutic surgery these costs might come to as much as $840 to $2,500 depending on the circumstances. And for adjuvant therapy, including periods of indisposition following treatment, one might have to add another $800 to $2,500.

Other costs such as transportation and special clothing might legitimately be counted. But, as mentioned early, these are not very large and can be subsumed in previously characterized costs for time expenditures for the sake of analysis.

PSYCHOSOCIAL COSTS

Psychologists, economists, and even the medical profession raise the issue of psychosocial costs to patients in discussions of the consequences of disease and therapy. The perspectives are usually different, with the medical

TABLE B.2

Estimated Procedural Costs for Detection and Diagnosis

Item	Cost range (dollars)	
	Washington University	BCDDP No. 25
History taking by paraprofessional[a]	10–25	
Clinical palpation and visual examination	40–60	
Mammography, including radiologist's fee	50–110	40
Thermography, including radiologist's fee	40–60	
Incisional or excisional biopsy, including hospital, medical, and pharmacy charges	500–1,000	n.a.[b]

n.a. = not applicable.

[a]Histories are ordinarily taken as an integral part of a clinical examination. It is listed separately here so as to account more precisely for its cost and the true cost of the clinical examination. Note that breast palpation may be done in the context of a gynecological examination and be billed at a lower rate.

[b]BCDDPs screen only. Recommended biopsies are done at a hospital selected by a woman and her personal physician. The entire screening process costs about $40 per visit.

Note: Other financial costs include hospital per diem, as appropriate, plus personal expenses of about $120 per day.

TABLE B.3
Estimated Procedural Costs for Therapy

Item	Cost Range (dollars)[a]
Unilateral mastectomy[b]	
Segmental	1,000–2,000
Simple	3,000–3,500
Radical and modified radical	3,500–5,200
Adjuvant therapy: chemo- and radiation therapy	
Breast reconstruction	3,000–5,000
Recurrence[c]	4,000–6,000

[a]All numbers are rounded to the nearest $100.

[b]This includes hospital, medical, surgical, and pharmacy charges as well as follow-up visits. Bilateral surgery does not necessarily double costs.

[c]Recurrence occurs in more than 50 percent of all cases within 10 years of surgery. Surgery, chemo- and radiation therapy may be utilized.

Note: Other financial costs include hospital per diem plus personal expenses of about 120 dollars/day.

profession emphasizing potential gains from early detection and treatment, psychologists often focusing on individual trauma, and economists usually concentrating on societal aspects of such costs. While the presence of psychosocial costs is widely appreciated, attempts to estimate their magnitudes in dollar-equivalent terms are rare.

Clark C. Abt, working with John P. Bunker, Frederick Mosteller, and others at Harvard in the late 1970s developed a list of psychosocial costs appropriate to breast cancer cases and estimated corresponding dollar values in terms of appropriate market prices reflecting the worth of opportunities missed by patients and their immediate families [Abt 1977]. He noted that suicide rates and the need for psychiatric care were somewhat higher among breast cancer patients. Adding all associated costs, he obtained a conservative estimate of about $3,000 per year. To account for pain and suffering he added costs of drugs and physician visits ($1,000 per year) to reduced job efficiency ($1,800). To account for family impacts he added counseling costs to reduce family conflict, which appears to be more common in such cases ($1,000), to annualized long-term earnings foregone by offspring due to disrupted child development, which is more common in families or widowed fathers ($3,100). These can be converted to present-equivalent values by the methods outlined in Chapter 5.[4]

Abt also tallied psychosocial costs directly related to breast amputation. These included psychological and medical treatment for such things as grief at the loss of a body part, worry over disfigurement and recurrence, and pain; inconvenience of hospitalization; and limitations on work and recreation, sexual relations, and other aspects of quality of life. The total came to $30,500 (present-equivalent dollars), assuming that women having a mastectomy live three years longer than those who do not.

These estimates are certainly not excessive. In reading Abt's analysis one is struck with the reasonableness of each of the individual costs. Even a doubling or tripling of these estimates would not seem unreasonable for some of the major items.

There are psychosocial costs related to a negative biopsy as well. These can be reconstructed in part from Abt's other estimates. One would get $8,000 to $10,000. From a different perspective Eddy [1980] reported that the psychosocial cost associated with the surgical scar alone, determined by direct questioning of women, ranges from practically nothing to $10,000. All of these estimates are tallied in Table B.4.

TABLE B.4
Estimated Psychosocial Costs

Item	Original Estimate (dollars)	Scaled to 1981 Dollars[a]
Increased suicide rates, psychotherapy drugs, and physician visits among close relatives—annualized costs[b]	4,000	5,450
Disrupted child development and its economic and social impacts—present-equivalent costs[a]	3,100	4,200
Reduced work efficiency of the patient from all related causes whether as a homemaker or as an employee—annualized costs[c]	1,800	2,450
Costs directly related to breast amputation: pain, impact on sex life, limitation on active work and on recreation, psychotherapy for worry about disfigurement and possible recurrence, and other aspects of reduced quality of life—present-equivalent costs	10,500	14,280
Impact of surgical scar from negative biopsy—present-equivalent cost of all aspects	10,000	10,000

[a]Costs are scaled to approximate 1981 dollar values using an 8 percent growth factor.

[b]Abt presumably envisioned these costs being incurred for three to six years, assuming, as he did, that patients undergoing mastectomy live for five years on the average, while others live for only two years. Current data indicate that the expected lifetime of mastectomy patients may be as high as 10 years if the disease is caught in an early stage. We presume these costs are incurred annually for up to 10 years and that all breast cancer victims have a mastectomy.

[c]These are based on the difference in lifetime earnings of college versus high school graduates ($3,000 per year) and are adjusted slightly ($100 per year) to reflect increased delinquency rates.

Note: All estimates are from Abt [1977] except that for the impact of surgical scar from negative biopsy, which is from Eddy [1981].

VALUING A HUMAN LIFE

The whole purpose of early detection and treatment is to extend life. If a life had no value, one would not expend other scarce resources to extend it. The fact that we expend vast resources as individuals and as a society to extend lives or reduce the chance of untimely death from accidents, murder, and so forth—is powerful evidence that we place a high value on human life.

Humans have struggled with the problem of valuing a human life since the beginning of written history, at least. Economists as professionals have been struggling with it for centuries [Fein 1976]. They are nowhere near a solution to this perplexing problem, but they do have some substantial insights into the issues surrounding various methods of value estimation. Because of their work, we can at least assign some ranges of value for analytical purposes.

The main approaches to assigning a dollar-equivalent value to life extension are discussed eloquently by Zeckhauser [1975] and Mishan [1976]. Three frequently proposed economic approaches are discounted consumption (lost because of early death), discounted production, and an individual's net dollar contribution to society. These are commonly bundled into a group labeled human capital approaches. The major objections to these approaches are that nonmonetary aspects like the mere pleasure of living are ignored. More important, none is a measure of either an individual's or society's willingness to pay to extend lives, yet willingness to pay is the fundamental economic concept applicable to economic choice.

Less frequently used, but potentially more valid, approaches are direct assessments of willingness to pay for risk reduction, and calculation of implied life value from pay differentials to workers in risky jobs. Acton [1976] conducted a survey to determine how much people would pay for mobile cardiac units to reduce the probability of their death from a heart attack. The responses yielded not unreasonable averages of about $28,000 for risk reduction of 1/1000 and $43,000 for risk reduction of 1/500. Thaler and Rosen estimated that workers in risky jobs valued their lives at about $200,000, a seemingly modest sum except that there is reason to believe that such workers often value their lives less than individuals not in such positions. [See Zeckhauser 1975.] In 1963 Carlson estimated that flight pay for air force captains suggested a life value of $135,000 to $980,000. [See Zeckhauser 1975.] Abt [1977] observed that court settlements for 10 to 30 years of reduced life often range from $200,000 to $300,000. Recent seetlements by Ford Motor Company pertaining to Pinto explosions have been closer to $1 million for 20 years of life lost. And recent medical malpractice settlements have exceeded $3 million for morbid events alone [St. Louis *Post Dispatch* 1981].

The many technical and logical difficulties inherent in those estimation approaches are discussed at length by Zeckhauser [1975]. We have already mentioned a few. We will not cover them all, but two additional issues are worth mentioning here. First, context strongly influences valuations. People faced with certain, possibly imminent, death from some cause, unless something is done to prevent it, are willing to pay far more for prevention than are those facing only a remote threat from the causal agent. Those facing, say, a 30 percent chance of early death from agent A are not likely to be very concerned about an increased risk of 0.1 percent from agent B. And constraints on financial resources influence willingness to pay. Second, willingness to pay to avoid risk must account for anxiety, which accompanies the mere awareness of risk. It is not clear how the level of anxiety relates to the level of risk on the average, let alone for individuals who may be more or less risk averse in their perspectives.

Table B.5 summarizes the value-of-life estimates discussed. All the numbers have been scaled up to reflect an average annual rate of increase of about 8 percent. None of those estimates can be considered accurate. Their primary value is in providing some reasonable bounds on the value of a human life as a basis for analytical investigations.

TABLE B.5
Value-of-Life Estimates by Various Researchers (in dollars)

Method	Age at Death (years)	
	45	50
Human capital[a]		
Undiscounted sum of lifetime earnings expected less future maintenance	250,000	175,000
Discounted (8 percent) future earnings expected less future maintenance	123,000	111,300
Willingness to pay for risk reduction		
Workers in risky jobs	300,000	2,400,000
Heart attack victims[b]		
1/1,000 reduction	49,000	49,000
1/500 reduction	60,000	60,000
Court settlements per year of life lost[c,d]	15,000	70,000
Malpractice—indefinitely comatose as opposed to death[d,e]	3,400,000	—

[a]Assuming an annual net income of $15,000, expected life in the absence of the immediate cause of untimely death is 76 years, retirement at age 65 is standard, and nursing home residence begins at 72 years of age and costs $10,000 annually.

[b]See Acton 1976.

[c]Zeckhauser 1975.

[d]As much as 38 to 45 percent of a settlement goes for lawyer and court cost [Reder 1978].

[e]St. Louis *Post Dispatch* 1981.

Note: Values are scaled to approximate 1981 dollars.

RADIATION RISK

Each rad of radiation carries with it a carcinogenic risk of 3.5 to 7.5 × 10⁻⁶ cancers per year for life beginning 10 years after irradiation. These are cancers that would not otherwise have developed and carry very high opportunity costs. Using $2 million as the opportunity cost of such a

TABLE B.6
Summary of Baseline Cost Estimates Specific to the Decision Maker (in dollars)

Category	Cost to	
	Patient	**Third-Party Payer**
Early detection[a]		n.a.
History	10–25	n.a.
Clinical exam	40–60	n.a.
Mammography	50–110	n.a.
Thermography	40–60	n.a.
Biopsy	n.a.	500–1,000
Treatment[b]		
Segmental	n.a.	1,000–2,000
Simple	n.a.	3,000–5,000
Radical	n.a.	3,500–5,200
Adjuvant	n.a.	1,000–2,000
Recurrence	n.a.	3,000–5,000
Breast reconstruction[c]	3,000–5,000	n.a.
Psychosocial[d]		
Negative biopsy	10,000–12,500	n.a.
Segmental mastectomy	20,000–25,000	n.a.
Simple mastectomy	35,000–45,000	n.a.
Radical mastectomy	39,000–50,000	n.a.
Value of life[e]	500,000–3,000,000	n.a.

n.a. = not available.

[a]Ordinarily, patients pay for breast examinations. Third-party payers can investigate the virtues of paying these costs.

[b]Unilateral breast disease is assumed. Bilateral mastectomy costs about 25 percent more. Segmental mastectomy, like negative biopsy, requires three to four days of hospitalization. Simple and radical mastectomy require 10 to 15 days of hospitalization, on the average.

[c]Breast reconstruction may require multiple hospitalizations. A major fraction of the costs is borne by the patient.

[d]These are present-equivalent values of costs occurring over an extended period. The average lifetime for breast cancer patients with successful treatment appears to be about 5–10 years [Shapiro et al. 1974]. The costs for radical mastectomy are from Abt [1977]. Costs for less severe surgery are scaled down nonlinearly.

[e]These are maximum values. We postulate that humans value their lives at a near constant level that depreciates only slowly with time as various other factors compete in that life [Gohagan and Swift, 1981]. This is a distinctly different concept than the human capital idea used by many others.

cancer, we calculate about 5 to 10 dollar-equivalents per Xerox mammogram per year beginning 10 years after the examination [Gohagan et al. 1981]. (Dollar-equivalent costs for low-dose mammograms of equal quality would be less.) Thus, 30 years after mammogram, the accumulated cost is about $200 to $300 dollars per woman screened.

SUMMARY

Some of the costs itemized in this chapter we know fairly accurately from hospital data. Of psychological costs that are even more central to decision making we have only rough approximations. The latter are costs we cannot measure directly, and we must fall back on the experience of other researchers for initial approximations. But even with all the uncertainty in many of the cost factors, we now have a reasonable basis upon which to begin analyses of decision alternatives (strategies and schedules). And, it turns out, more accurate estimates are not essential to our ultimate recommendations.

The numerical cost ranges used as starting values for the analyses are summarized in Table B.6 for the separate perspectives of patients and third-party payers.

NOTES

1. All three methods assign values to a human life by age. The implications of these methods are discussed below from an economic perspective. They are discussed elsewhere from a screening perspective where all three methods are rejected in favor of a constant value for adult human lives, which declines only late in life, according to life tables reflecting multiple competing factors for a life [Gohagan and Swift 1981].

2. Ultrasonics represents another possible detection modality. However, it is almost certainly not yet at the stage of development where it can be depended on to detect either neoplasms less than a centimeter in diameter or tiny microcalcifications associated with malignancy. It is better suited to differentiation between small fluid-filled cysts and solid masses once a mass has been identified by some other modality. In addition, we have no detection data on ultrasonics from our own screening effort, so that ultrasonics cannot be empirically evaluated against the other modalities in our analyses.

3. Eddy [1981] asked a very cautious woman who had Pap smears done annually what she thought that episode cost her. She responded that she would be glad to relinquish $100 in lieu of the examination and all the prearrangements that accompany it. Although there are other factors in addition to direct financial costs covered in this woman's response, the procedure clearly costs far more than merely an office-plus-test fee.

4. In 1853 William Farr estimated the worth of a human at any age as the sum of future expected wages less the sum of future maintenance. The idea was that much capital is invested in the development of a productive human and subsequent care of older persons. This investment was to be balanced by earnings, or return on the investment over time. Economists now discount these cash flows to reflect limited present worth of future flows when they employ this method.

REFERENCES

Abt CC (1977) The issue of social costs in cost-benefit analysis of surgery, *in* Bunker JP, Barnes BA, Mosteller F (eds), Costs, risks, and benefits of surgery. New York, Oxford University Press.

Acton JP (1976) Measuring the monetary value of lifesaving programs. Law and Contemporary Próblems 40:46-72.

Bayles MD (1978) The price of life. Ethics 80:20-34.

Calabresi G, Babbitt P (1978) Tragic choices. New York, W. W. Norton.

Drummond MF (1980) Principles of economic appraisal in health care. New York Oxford University Press.

Eddy DM (1981) The economics of cancer prevention and detection: getting more for less. Cancer 47:1200-1209.

Eddy DM (1980) Screening for cancer: theory analysis and design. Englewood Cliffs, N.J., Prentice-Hall.

Fein R (1976) On measuring economic benefits of health programs, *in* Veatch RM, Branson R (eds). Ethics and health policy. Cambridge, Mass., Ballinger.

Gohagan JK, Spitznagel EL, Darby WP, Feiner JB (1981) Optimal strategies for breast cancer detection. Proceedings of the International Conference on Systems Science in Health Care. New York, Pergamon Press.

Gohagan JK, Swift JG (1981) Scheduling Pap smears for asymptomatic women. Preventive Medicine 10:741-753.

McPeek B, Gilbert JP, Mosteller F (1976) The end result: quality of life, *in* Bunker JP, Barnes BA, Mosteller F (eds), Costs, risks, and benefits of surgery. New York, Oxford Univeristy Press.

Mishan EJ (1976) Cost-benefit analysis. New York, Praeger.

Reder MW (1978) Contingent fees in litigation with special reference to medical malpractice, *in* Rottenberg S (ed), The economics of medical malpractice. Washington, D.C., American Enterprise Institution for Public Policy Research.

Shapiro S, Strax P, Venet L, Venet W (1974) Changes in 5-year breast cancer mortality in a breast cancer screening program, *in* Seventh National Cancer Conference Proceedings, pp. 663-678. New York, American Cancer Society, January 1974.

St. Louis Post Dispatch (1981) Comatose woman awarded $3 million, April 5, 1981, p. 5A.

Vorherr H (1980) Breast cancer: epidemiology, endocrinology, biochemistry and pathology. Baltimore-Munich, Urban and Schwarzenberg.

Zeckhauser R (1975) Procedures for valuing lives. Public Policy 23:419-464.

Zeckhauser R, Shepard D (1976) Where now for saving lives? Law and Contemporary Problems 40:5-45.

Index